Exercise:

Get Fit Fast Working Smarter Not Harder - Lose Weight, Strength, Workout & Weight Training

Table of Contents

Bonus

As my passion is sharing valuable information that tangibly impacts your life, I'd like to invite you to the free bonus below to positively affect your life in other dimensions, along with other tried and true methods I will send you.

If you want to take your health to the next level, I recommend the free resource below for some easy-to-follow quick tips that make a huge impact. ***If you sign up, you will get the bonus immediately sent to your <u>valid</u> email address.***

Check the link below:

https://publishfs.leadpages.co/getultrahealth/

23 Health Tips & Hacks You Probably Aren't Doing But Should Be to Reduce Fatigue, Improve Sleep and Recovery, Boost Sex Drive, and Heal Your Gut

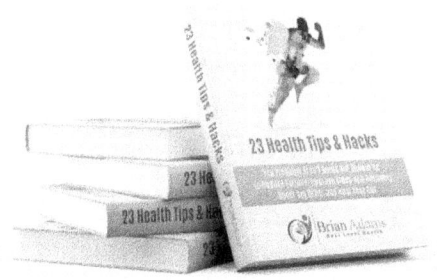

Introduction

The age-old adage that "Health is Wealth" has been used and re used umpteen number of times, but the yet the true essence of what that simple string of words try to convey cannot be stressed enough. The great Herophiles captured the stark truth and laid it bare before us when he said the words that I had quoted in the beginning,

If we pause for a moment and reflect on what he has said, it is indeed so apparent that the revelation brings a pang of shame to our mind that is tough to gulp down. Lack of goof mental and physical health can cripple our lives in many more ways than we imagine. It can blunt our intellectual prowess, can break us physically, smother our existence with ailments and diseases, and simply take the joy and meaning out of living.

In fact, the most alarming development is that millions and millions of people continue to conduct their lives while staying immersed in the seas of oblivion. But that is completely fine when you discover that an equal if not larger number of people are actually aware of this fact but still are apprehensive to emerge out of the fake cocoon of happiness that they have enveloped themselves with. They fail to accept the truth that is staring at their faces, choosing instead to turn away and consoling themselves that what they are doing is the "right" or the "normal" thing to do.

Over the last few years, words like fitness, health, diets, gym, workouts etc have become a mainstay of our lives and conversations. It was not like this a decade ago. Back then, relatively few people could afford machines to do their work for them and make their lives easier. Look back at the era of your grandparents and parents. They did almost everything by hand. Washing clothes, chopping vegetables, kneading flour, baking bread, traveling long distances on foot, carrying heavy things from one place to another. In rural areas, women would get up early and walk many kilometers to fetch water. Threshing, winnowing, harvesting, farming- everything was done manually. People back then used the so-called compound movements of today, like the squat, overhead press and deadlift, to carry out normal, day-to-day activities. No wonder then, that their generation was so darn fit! If you observe the age of dying in that generation, save for some neonatal or environmental factors, almost everyone used to be hale, hearty and fit even when they were well into their nineties, with excellent teeth, hair, skin, circulation, digestion and overall health.

What's happening now?

Everywhere you look, you see young people, in their early twenties and thirties succumbing to a host of lifestyle diseases. Diabetes, hypertension, high blood pressure, kidney problems, mental stress, obesity, and a sedentary lifestyle - these were almost unheard of in the last decade. Owing to the rapid change in the job environment, young people are now earning almost eight to ten times more than their parents used to, but they also have an immense amount of stress to deal with. To combat that, instead of looking at healthier alternatives like walking or playing with their children or climbing stairs every day, they indulge in eating junk food, to comfort their stressed out minds. This, combined with dangerous levels of inactivity, has led to an alarming increase in lifestyle diseases. People no longer want to wait for a period of time before they can see results in their workout regime. They want instant results. Most of them either resort to mindless cardio and aerobic workouts or indulge in the latest diet fads in the market. But none of these methods works for a long time and ultimately, they pay the price with their poor and patchy health.

I say this not because I wish to be called the harbinger of doomsday, but because the number of people who relegate health and fitness to the least important sphere of their lives constitute the vast majority amongst us.

One of the primary reasons for this is the pace of life in these turbulent times. People seldom find the time to devote to anything other than their vocations and the incessant race to reach the top. But the simple question remains as to what is the point of racing to the summit if you are going to collapse at the top out of the breathless exertion that you have put your bodies through.

As I mentioned above, this less-than-favorable outlook towards exercise is because of the misconceptions associated with it. Partly spread by people who never tried exercising and partly by those who did try, but in the wrong way. And that is precisely what I intend to set straight with this book. Because I firmly believe in the notion that if done the right way, exercise and fitness can truly transform your life beyond your farthest expectations. The benefits would not be felt just in terms of physical health, but in every other significant avenue of your life.

This book is divided into seven chapters. The first chapter is where I shall touch upon the basic concept of exercising in the smart way as against the hard way (mind you; there is a lot of difference between the two!). The second chapter covers the whole concept of aerobic exercise. In the third chapter I will be covering the basic principles of weight training including the theoretical and practical ethos of this discipline. The fourth and fifth chapters deal with compound and isolation exercises. High Intensity Interval Training and CrossFit Training are dealt with in the next two chapters and a final chapter is devoted to diet and nutrition.

I thank you for purchasing this book and hope that you find it useful.

Chapter 1: Work Out Smart

The fact needs to be reiterated that the prime reason for people not taking up exercise and physical fitness regularly are the multitudes of misconceptions and malafide information associated with it. And the reason for the quitters is the hardship they have to go through on a daily basis. It will be correct for you to assume that in this chapter I intend to address both of these issues.

First and foremost, let us establish without doubt that, done with the right frame of mind, exercise can very be the most gratifying part of your whole day. As I had mentioned before, the benefits of that half an hour or one hour spent exercising can spill over to the rest of the day and actually play a huge role in making you feel positive.

The second important thing is the notion that makes people quit; that is the hatred of the exercises and other practices they do in order to remain fit. The remedy to this problem is extremely simple yet extremely effective. All you need to do is love what you do. Do not look upon the time spent every day on the treadmill or in the gym as a session of torture; instead consider it as the time of physical invigoration and emancipation. When you love an activity, the difficulties endured in performing that activity turn to enjoyable challenges that inspire to push yourself.

The key to satisfying both these criterion lies in a simple revamping of your perception. What needs to be changed is the age-old way of thinking that physical exercise is something that needs to be hard in order to be effective.

But as Bob Dylan sang, in what now feels to be an eon ago, times are changing and that means so should your thought process. Scientists and researchers have proved it beyond doubt that the physical exercise needs to be smart rather than merely hard.

Now, don't even imagine for a second that there is some hot shot new technology by which you just need to scamper around a few steps and lift a couple of extra-light dumbbells to stay ship shape. No that's not what I meant by the term "working out smart". What that phrase means is that you need to ask yourself certain questions and try answering them in the most honest way. The following are the questions:

1. Do I really love and enjoy the practice of regular exercise? If not, then why?
2. What is my primary objective?
3. Is my exercise regimen really effective? If not, then what can I do in order to improve the efficacy?
4. How can I make my workouts smarter?

These are the four questions that I shall be covering in this chapter. This is very important because before we go in depth into the various technicalities of weight training and aerobics etc., we must first get the basics right. So let us tackle the questions one by one

Do I really love exercising?

The underlying intention behind asking yourself this question is very simple, and yet so important. It is an inherent basic human nature that we can only do something effectively and efficiently if we really love it.

Any action done begrudgingly will deliver only sub-par results. This principle holds true in all areas of our life, be it professional or personal. And there is no reason why it should not apply to your physical fitness regimen as well.

In any kind of physical exercise, be it aerobics or weight training or any other ancillary form, you whole hearted dedication is an unavoidable requisite. And thus dedication stems from your love for that activity. There is a reason why I have stressed upon this and we shall take a look at that with the help of weight training as an example. Weight training is hard; there is no doubt about that. And it shall be effective only if you push yourself hard. If you can curl 30 pounds with your arms, then development will occur only if you manage to lift heavier consistently. And that mental conviction to push your body physically will only come from the love and dedication within you. And hence the importance of asking yourself whether you love exercising or not. Because if you don't, then somehow inspire yourself to living healthy by taking up regular physical exercise.

What is my primary objective?

Having looked at the first question, let us move on to the second one. This is where you ask yourself what exactly is your primary objective behind exercising. This question holds an immense amount of significance because like anything else in your life, the route you take depends on the objective you have fixed for yourself. Similarly, the methodology of your exercise will depend on what you are aiming for. For instance, the exercise regimen of a person training for a 20-mile marathon will be very different from that of a wrestler or boxer. Both are as drastically different from each other as they can be.

Hence you have to ascertain whether your objective is a long term one or a short term one. You have to decide whether you consider physical fitness as a life-long objective or whether you are pursuing a more short term goal such as preparing yourself for a competition or meet. Because, as I said earlier, in order for your exercise regimen to be smart and effective, it should be tweaked to meet the requirements of your objective. Hence it is very apparent that it is extremely important to arrive at your objectives with as much clarity as possible because as I have said, lack of a solid objective is the biggest hindrance to achieving efficiency in your workouts.

How can I make my exercise regimen more effective?

Asking yourself this question will be much more easy than the previous two questions. Because of the simple reason that by answering the first two questions you have made sure that you are indeed on the right path with the right intention. Two kinds of people would have reached this stage in a satisfactory manner. The first group would be the beginners, who wish to adopt a lifestyle of physical fitness. The second group would be those are already engaged in some kind of physical activity on a regular basis.

But the present question holds value whether you belong to the first group or the second one. It is one thing to be engaging yourself in some kind physical activity on a regular basis, while it is a completely different thing to go about your workouts in the most efficient method possible. This intended increase in efficiency calls for a proper self-appraisal. I say this is important because this is one area where your own rating of your performance matters much higher than that of others.

After asking yourself this question, you have to reflect on the matter and find out the lacunae. Sniff out where you are lacking. There are many factors here, some apparent, while some others may not be so obvious. Your exercise regimen may be lacking in terms of correct technique of movements or insufficient nutrition or rest or even lack of motivation. When it comes to technique and principles of exercise I shall covering them I detail in the forthcoming chapters. But it is imperative that you ascertain where your efficiency can be improved.

How can I make my workouts smarter?

This is the core subject of this book and hence demands the maximum attention in this regard. The idea is to figure out how you can make your workouts smarter. The phrase "smarter" used here has a wide scope as it covers much more than its literal meaning. As I had mentioned earlier, the most important aspect is to work out smart and not merely hard. Simply because of the fact that a lot of hard work done in a blind fashion will yield much lesser results than the similar amount of work done in the smart way.

"Smart" here signifies aspects like the correct number of repetitions, the right number of sets of an exercise, the apt duration of rest time between sets, lifting the ideal amount of weights for each body part depending on whether the intention is gain of strength or endurance or size, the right amount of aerobics, the number of meals a day and the pattern, so on and so forth. As you can see here, the word "smart" encompasses a very wide array of parameters and notions that all have to looked at.

Many of these factors are major ones that have a prominent impact on your exercise regimen. The benefits of these are immediately noticeable. Some factors may not have that radical an impact but over a period of time you will begin to see the results. In the subsequent chapters we will go over these factors one by one in depth.

But first, let us see what the hue and cry about fitness is all about.

What Exactly Is Fitness?

Fitness in a nutshell, is all about being able to carry out your day-to-day activities with ease and minimal strain. Fitness is a state of overall well being. Just because you are able to lift 200 pounds at the gym does not mean anything if you begin gasping for breath after climbing two flights of stairs. Gym and fitness of course, go hand in hand, but fitness is more, so much more than just a workout at the gym. In this age, when everyone is suddenly health conscious, gyms are becoming overcrowded. You hardly find any free machines or the proper weights, plus with work becoming more and more complicated, it is definitely a hassle to find a proper gym, get there at a decent hour before the rush, complete your workout and come back home. Bodyweight training is a lifesaver in this regard. You can train in the privacy of your home, for as long or as little you want to. You get to decide how much you want to do on a particular day. The question is not whether you decide to hit the gym or do bodyweight or dedicate yourself to yoga or calisthenics. Fitness is a lifelong state of mind-body equilibrium.

What Fitness Is Not? Myths Regarding Fitness and Training

Just like diet and nutrition, there are tons of misconceptions regarding fitness. Some of them are listed below:

• I can spot reduce the fat in my abdomen-

People believe with all their heart that doing a hundred crunches and fifty situps will magically reduce the fat around their midsection. Spot reduction is a myth. When you lose fat, you lose it from your entire body, not just one part. That is possible only when you undergo liposuction.

• Fat people are unhealthy-

Fitness and flexibility have nothing to do with your size. A person who looks bulky and fat might be far healthier than a person who looks slim and thin.

• You can eat what you want-

Just because you hit the gym does not mean you come back home and load up on junk food and unhealthy meals. All your good work will come undone if you keep up this habit.

- Your metabolism slows down after you hit 30-

There's no scientific basis for this sentence. Your metabolism gets hit negatively due to a combination of genetic factors, hormones and inactivity. If you don't eat healthy and get regular exercise, you will get out of shape no matter what age you are.

- You can't gain muscle after you are 40-

You can gain muscle at any point you want to- but yes, as we age, we do need to get ourselves checked by a doctor. If you're in reasonably good physical condition, with no life threatening ailments to boot, there's no reason why you cannot embark on a fitness journey.

- The more you sweat, the more fat you lose-

Sweating is the body's response to the cooling mechanism it activates when the inner temperature increases. It is simply a matter of homeostasis. Fat loss has nothing to do with how much you sweat.

- No pain, no gain-

Most gym goers ardently believe that if their workout wasn't brutal, if their muscles aren't sore the next day, they haven't trained hard enough. That's not true. If you've reached your fitness goal for the day or week, it does not matter whether or not you're sore the next day.

• I need to spend a minimum of two hours in the gym every day-

You're simply wasting your time. A workout should be effective and hit the maximum number of muscle groups. You can just as easily be done within 50 minutes, if you incorporate compound movements like the squat, deadlift and bench press, instead of putting in one hour's worth of bicep curls.

• I need to confuse my muscles so all of them get an equal workout-

This is a favourite amongst gym goers- to confuse their body and muscle groups by engaging in a variety of exercises each day. This is plain stupid. The body is much smarter than we are. All we need to do is hit the maximum body parts and joints with the minimum of movements and repeat them day in and day out. Boring is good, when it comes to fitness.

• Machines are much safer than free weights-

People, especially women, fear free weights more than any other piece of gym equipment. They will spend hours on the treadmill, the cable push down machine, the leg press, the Smith machine, but will not venture near the barbells and dumbbells. This is unfortunate. Free weights and bars will give you more range of motion and complement the natural curve of your body as it does the movements. You might risk severe injury on the machines and not even be aware of it.

People also feel that they aren't doing enough for their bodies if they don't hit the gym. Fitness is not just about running on the treadmill or lifting weights or beating your PR. A brisk walk, climbing stairs, running with your children, playing ball, walking the dog, painting your house, gardening with your spouse, carrying furniture- all these are daily activities which will keep you fit and happy throughout your life. Great if you can join a gym and begin weight training, but don't be too upset about not being able to do it. Find your own rhythm, your own regime and your happiness. Fitness is not just about your body, but mind as well.

Chapter 2: Weight Loss 101- Aerobics

As you have already noticed, there are two main subjects dealt with in this book. One is weight loss and the other one is weight training. The objective is to study how you can enhance the efforts you take in each aspect by making the workouts smarter. In this chapter, we shall cover the two most important principles of weight loss; namely aerobics and diet. In fact, I would call these two concepts as the main pillars of weight loss. This is because efficient reduction of weight is possible only when you pair the right amount of aerobic exercises with the correct pattern of diet.

This is an area that is most overlooked by people. Many do it inadvertently because they may be oblivious to these basic principles of physical fitness. Others overlook these factors because they may be under the impression satisfying any one criterion will balance out the lack of another one. For instance, some consider working out in a strenuous fashion on a regular basis while completely overlooking the significance of maintaining proper diet as a healthy practice.

Whatever be the case, the fact remains irrefutable that if losing that extra weight and staying lean is the objective then efficient and nutritious diet rides in tandem with regular and effective aerobic exercises. There is in fact a thumb rule that in order to stay lean and healthy, your diet and exercise should be in perfect ratio. This ratio takes into consideration the amount of calories you take through your food and the amount of calories you burn by means of physical exercise. Your body will maintain a lean physique if the amount of calories consumed in a day is more or less equal to or slightly more than the amount the calories spent in a day.

This pretty much means that your complete lifestyle will undergo a change for the better. This twin headed endeavor of pairing proper exercise with a healthy and nutrient rich diet would necessitate you to adopt a disciplined daily routine that eschews any ill habits. But the best part about this is that you would have umpteen permutations and combinations when it comes to mixing and matching your exercise modules and diet structure in order to avoid boredom. This is very important because a monotonous and boring routine is the biggest reason why people quit exercising. For instance, you could chalk out a schedule whereby you run the morning for three days a week and on the alternate days you would be doing stationary aerobics at home. This would go a long way in livening up your workouts.

Aerobics

In this section we shall be looking mainly at three key aspects; the basic principles of aerobic exercises and how to infuse an element of smartness into them, the benefits of performing aerobic exercises and some of the most effective aerobic exercises. So let us get started.

The basic principles:

Before we go into the actual aerobic exercises, let us first go over the basic principles of aerobic exercises. This is very important because if you are clear with the underlying concepts, then it will aid you immensely in improving the efficiency of your workouts and even modifying or customizing the various workouts to suit your requirements.

In the simplest sense of the word, aerobic exercise means any physical activity that depends on the free availability of oxygen as fuel for the activity. The process is called aerobic metabolism. What happens here is, during physical exertion, the glycogen in the body is broken down into the constituent glucose. This glucose that is produced undergoes a reaction called glycolysis. The by-product of this reaction is pyruvate. The oxygen that has entered the blood stream reacts with the pyruvate in a further reaction called Krebs cycle. This is an extremely complicated reaction about which we need not go into depth. The end result of the Krebs cycle is the production of energy.

You may have noticed by now that oxygen is the fulcrum of this whole system. But what happens when there is insufficient oxygen in the blood stream or when the pace of the exercise performed is too fast for the body to keep in pace? The resultant situation is called the anaerobic reaction. As I mentioned earlier, aerobic exercises make use of oxygen to fuel muscle contraction. Whereas in case of anaerobic exercises, other cellular reactions used to aid muscular contraction. These reactions do not rely on the availability of oxygen in the blood stream.

The result of anaerobic reactions is that in addition to production of energy, the body also produces something called lactate. When the intensity of the exercise becomes higher, the amount of lactate produced and stored in the body also becomes higher. The most apparent indication of lactate build-up in the muscles is the pain that we associate with muscular fatigue. When the intensity of the exercise is not reduced, then more and more lactate is stored in the muscles, thereby increasing the pain and burning sensation in the muscles.

Extreme manifestations of build up of lactate include nausea, fainting and vomiting. On the other hand, when the intensity of the work out is reduced, the body gradually removes the lactate that has accumulated in the muscles. All forms of high intensity exercises belong to the category of anaerobic exercises. For example, fast sprinting for short distances, and weigh training for size gains or strength improvements are classic instances of anaerobic exercises.

From what is mentioned above, it is quite clear that the aerobic exercises are physical activities that are performed at a level of intensity that is comparatively moderate, and for a period of time that is quite long in duration. These are in fact the most distinctive traits of aerobic exercises. There are many exercises or activities that satisfy the above said criteria, for example, long distance running or jogging at a sedate pace, stretching exercises, push ups at a low count, sports such as non-competitive singles tennis, rowing, trekking etc.

We can even reach at a conclusion that some sports and activities are inherently aerobic while some others are out and out anaerobic. There are even examples where the same sport can be played at a variable tempo thereby changing the nature of the activity from aerobic to anaerobic. A good example is tennis. Singles tennis played at a non-competitive level can be termed as aerobic because of the fact that the motions are continuous and flowing in nature. Whereas in case of doubles tennis, the movements are quick and sporadic making it more anaerobic than aerobic.

Benefits of aerobic exercises

I believe by now you must be quite conversant with the basic principles of aerobic activities. You would be able to differentiate between what can be called as an aerobic activity and what would be termed as anaerobic.

At this point we can have a look at what are the various benefits of aerobic exercise performed regularly.

- The most beneficial aspect of aerobic exercises is from the cardio vascular angle. It strengthens the heart tissues and improves the efficacy of the pumping action. Additionally, the blood vessels are also strengthened and this greatly diminishes the incidence of any circulatory disorders. Just like any other muscle tissue in the body, increased intensity of activity improves the vitality of the heart tissues as well.
- Enhancement of the efficacy of the pulmonary organs. This is another avenue where the benefits of aerobic activity shine through. The vital capacity of the lungs vastly improves with regular physical activity and exertion. And these benefits are not just

restricted to the capacity of the lungs alone. Whatever little risk of Bronchitis that you may have by reason of living in these polluted times, is negated by regular physical activity. This benefit is particularly seen in case of people who had been chain smokers and have quit only recently. In fact, it has been proved beyond doubt by virtue of the published results of many studies that regular and rigorous physical activity such as aerobics can be cathartic to lung tissue damage induced by smoking. It had been previously believed that the ill effects of smoking such as bronchitis and pulmonary tissue damage were irreversible. However complete abstinence paired with substantial physical exercise over the course of a decade can be so therapeutic that the lungs of such a person are virtually indistinguishable from that of a non-smoker in terms of the health of the tissues.

- There is no denying the fact that a healthy dose of aerobics on a daily basis goes a long way in boosting your mental acumen and prowess. This is due to the fact that the physical exertion that you undergo in order to perform aerobics and other similar activities entail in the release of many endorphins and other feel-good chemicals that plays a major role in lifting your mood. And such uplift is not restricted to the immediate few minutes after the exercise. Rather the effects are manifested throughout the day. All this means that the incidence of stress and stress related disorders would be reduced to the minimum. This holds particular significance in these times when mental depression is that Hydra can't be driven out in spite of repeated measures from our side. It is an omnipresent shadow waiting to butt its head into our lives. In such conditions, regular physical activity can prove to be the most efficient weapon in our quiver.

- Another mental benefit of aerobics is the increase in cognitive capacities and mental acumen. This is the reason why students are often advised to engage in some kind of aerobics such as running, swimming etc. on a regular basis.

- Aerobics and other physical activities also increase the oxygen carrying capacity of the blood. This happens because the production of Red Blood Cells is triggered.

- A reduction in the risk of developing lifestyle ailments such as Hypertension and Diabetes is only expected here. There is a reason why these diseases are called lifestyle diseases, and by engaging in regular physical exercise, you are drastically reducing the risk of such ailments by a huge degree. There are in fact countless studies by a number of reputed organizations that have established it beyond question that the regular exercise decreases the risk of diabetes by a great margin.

- Activities such as jogging and sports such as basketball have been shown as the perfect remedy for maintaining and increasing bone density, Children who are involved in these sports attain bone growth in a much healthier time frame than children who lead a sedentary lifestyle.

- I have saved the best and the most significant benefit (from the point of view of the subject handled by this book) for the last; weight loss. Obesity can very well be considered as the plague of our times, except that this plague is not bound by geographical or demographical boundaries. The benefits of regular practice of aerobics are indeed manifested the most when it comes to weight reduction. This is primarily because of the fact that the weight loss is something that cannot be achieved overnight. Nor is it something that can be retained effortlessly once achieved. Both these require diligent effort from your side that is not a short term one.

In order to tackle obesity people sometimes turn to varied number of techniques ranging from mediocre to outright bizarre. But research by scientists and nutrition specialists and true accounts from a huge number of people has established it beyond doubt that when it comes to weight reduction, no fancy diet or trick exercise machine can ever replicate or even come close to the efficacy of the aerobics and good diet.

- Till now we had been looking at only the health benefits of aerobics. But that is only half the cake. Aerobics has a multitude of performance-oriented benefits as well. This becomes more and more apparent in case of people engaged in active sports and other similar activities.

- One of the biggest advantages of aerobics is the boost in endurance that you get. Athletes the world over, regardless of the nature of sport, vouches for this fact. Be it a cricketer or a marathon runner, a wrestler or a tennis player, a footballer or a motorcycle racer, regular and diligent practice of aerobics provides them with increased endurance that is immensely vital to the sport, no matter what it is.

- Engaging in some kind aerobics on a daily basis also has an added benefit of decreasing the recovery period of muscles manifold. This is very important for athletes as well as non-athletes. The concept of recovery period is a very significant one that has far reaching consequences. Simply put, recovery period is the time taken by the muscles to recover from the injury from exertion. When I say the word "injury" I mean the micro tears in the muscle fibers as a result of constant contractions and extensions. This happens when you engage in some heavy workout or otherwise as well when you engage in some physical activity that your body is not used to. In such cases, you experience muscle soreness and pain and this can occur in varying degrees of severity. It has been proven that when you engage in aerobics on a regular basis, the time taken for your body to recover from these tears and other micro trauma decreases drastically.

Now that you have seen what are the basic principles of aerobic activities and the various benefits that you stand to enjoy, let us go over some of the key activities that come under the head aerobic exercises. I have compiled this list because confusion can very well arise as to whether some activity is aerobic or anaerobic in nature.

The activities or exercises can be broadly categorized, for the ease of comfort and understanding into activities that can be performed indoors as well as those that are done outdoors. The indoor activities include repeated climbing of stairs, rowing inside on a rowing machine, performing push ups, performing sit ups, running on a treadmill, skipping, stationary jogging, using a stationary bicycle, jumping jacks etc. The best thing about aerobic exercises is that unlike other forms of exercises, these can be done at any time and hence there is no strict code of conduct that has to be followed. As long as your methodology is correct and your form remains proper, you can pretty much infuse any amount of variation into your exercises.

The various aerobic activities that can be performed outdoors are a vast list that includes swimming, trekking, hiking, trail running, cycling, walking, playing sports etc.

Chapter 3: Weight Training

In the last chapter we saw the how regular aerobics and correct diet contribute towards helping you shed those extra kilos. This chapter will concentrate on the other key subject of this book: weight training. AS the name implies weight training is a form of exercise that makes use of free weights in the dumbbells and barbells and kettle balls and weight machines to build the strength and endurance muscular size of your body.

So, what exactly is weight training? Something only bulky bodybuilders do? How do you get started? What are the most effective exercises? What happens to our body when we strength train. Read on to find answers to these questions.

Weight training refers to providing the body with some form of resistance, mostly in the form of weights, either free weights or machine weights, in order to give pressure to the muscles and make them grow. You can spend hours on the treadmill or do a million aerobic exercises. Your heart becomes healthier, no doubt, but you will never gain those rippling muscles or that washboard flat abs with a six pack. To achieve that, strength training is the way to go.

The concept of weight training is age old one that can be traced to the earliest civilizations. It can even be said that the as long as the history of man and his roots has been written, some kind of reference to weight lifting and weight training has always found a mention. All kind of mythological stories are awash with stories and anecdotes of strong men and their feats.

Perhaps the earliest one is the story if the Greek wrestler Milo. As the legend goes, Milo was a famed wrestler in Greece. His strength and prowess were famous in all of the Greek states and beyond. No matter how much they practiced or trained, his fellow wrestlers could never better the strength and endurance of Milo. The secret of his seemingly superhuman strength lies in the weird habit that Milo had. When a cow in his home gave birth, milo immediately took to the calf in a very fond manner. He developed a habit of carrying the calf wherever he went.

The sight of Milo walking down the street with a calf slung over his powerful shoulders became such a common sight for the villagers that they soon started ignoring it. The calf became progressively bigger and heavier as time passed, but its placed was still on Milo's shoulders. This went on until the calf became a fully-grown adult cow and one fine day, he gave the cows to the butchers to be slaughtered. It does not end here, Milo is said to have eaten the whole cow himself.

However, smothered by hyperbole this story may be, we can't ignore two key concepts pertaining to weight training here. Because if this is not the best example of progressive resistance weight training and the importance of good protein rich diet, then I don't know what is. What Milo supposedly performed centuries ago is not much different in principle and practice from modern day weightlifters and bodybuilders do.

The basic concepts behind weight training are indeed quite simple. The process goes like this; when you train with free weights for a body part, let us say your arm, you lift the weights in a continuous motion for a predetermined number of repetitions. A fixed number of repetitions constitute a set of that exercise and you should be performing anything between four to ten sets. Let us assume that on the first day you perform four sets of Bicep Curls using twenty ponds. By the end of the fourth set, you would be really struggling to complete the set. Continue doing this for a week or two and by the end of the second week you would be lifting and curling the same weight in the fourth set with comparative ease. So what has happened here? Your own body that was huffing and puffing to complete four sets is now able to do six sets before giving up. What has happened here is a classic instance of progressive weight training.

Because of your consistent and regular weight training, your body became acclimatized to lifting twenty pounds. The muscle fibers in your arm, or more specifically your biceps sensed the fact that they have to lift twenty pounds every day, many times. And because of this progressive and constant stimuli, the strength and endurance in your arms increased.

After this when you increase the difficulty level of your exercise by increasing the weight or reducing the rest time between sets or by performing supersets (performing two different exercises, targeting two different muscle groups back to back), then you will undoubtedly experience difficulty in the beginning, But sticking to your plan and willing your body to perform again and again till failure will eventually take you to a day when you can lift that higher amount of weight or exercise with that reduced rest time, without failure. This adaptive capacity of the body is the underlying principle of weight training.

At this point you may be wondering where the "smart" angle comes into the picture. The simplicity of the underlying concepts of weight training is indeed akin to a twin edged sword. On one hand, this ease makes it convenient to grasp the ethos and makes the diligent and disciplined person less prone to mistakes. It lets you bring a great amount of variation into the exercise routine that will help you customize the workouts to suit your lifestyle.

On the other hand, an undisciplined practitioner, looking to find an easy way to increase the strength and size of his muscles may simply take the key concepts for granted. This is a very common mistake that people make and eventually they resort to sloppy techniques and poor form in performing exercises. This will, sooner than later result in injury and irreparable damage to the joints and ligaments that will be tough to recover from.

And this is precisely what I intend to address in the forthcoming sections of this chapter. Weight training is something that can provide you with immense amount of benefits if done in the right way. We will go a step further and do it the smart way. I will mention techniques and tips that you can adopt in order train efficiently and without the risk of injury. You can see how to train hard and smart not merely swing around some heavy dumbbells in the gym without a clue about what to do.

Why Should You Strength Train?

Increased EPOC-

Leave cardio aside. Strength training provides you with a much greater level of EPOC, excess post-exercise oxygen consumption. What's this? Well, your body years for equilibrium. After your workout, it desperately wants to get back to its original state. When you work with weights, this state of equilibrium is shattered. And the body uses a TON of energy and calorie burning process to get back to its original state. So, a win- win for everybody. Studies have shown that this EPOC or metabolism burning state is switched on for more than 40 hours after a bout of strength training.

Elevated RMR-

Your resting metabolic rate, that means, the rate at which you burn calories while resting, is also boosted by strength training. This is because your body burns more calories trying to replenish its torn muscles and fibers and this repairing process consumes a lot of calories and fuel from the body.

A Healthier You-

Hours of jumping and cardio will only make you tired. Strength training will not only strengthen your heart, it will also sculpt a strong core, build your legs, chest, back, improve circulation, improves muscle tone, balances your coordination and your overall health is much, much better.

Say goodbye to diseases-

When you begin weight training, you will find, to your utter astonishment, that all your minor ailments and illness go away and never bother you again. That's because of your increased level of immunity which strength training offers you. Not only this, serious conditions like heart disease, diabetes, high blood pressure etc. are also kept at bay with strength training, because it makes your heart and other body parts extremely strong and immune to outside pathogens.

Training for Strength, Endurance and Size:

There are three key objectives behind weight training; increase in strength, improvement in endurance and better aesthetics in the form of more size and enhanced definition among muscle groups. Any other objective will fall under these main objects as ancillary motives. Contrary to what many people think, it is extremely difficult or near impossible to achieve all three of these objectives simultaneously. There is a significant amount of difference in approach and technique as well. So let us look at these three methods in a little more detail

If your intention is increasing your general strength, then all the exercises you perform for various muscle groups should be done keeping three main points in mind. First of all, make sure that the weights you use are quite heavy. In fact, they should be heavy enough to not let you perform more than 4 or 5 repetitions in a set. The second point is the above mentioned number of repetitions in a single set of an exercise; make sure it is in the lower range (5 or 6 maximum). The third factor is the rest period between twos sets. Ensure that you take ample rest between two sets. The ideal range will be between 2 to 3 minutes.

The above-mentioned three factors apply in case of exercises performed with an intention to increase the endurance of your muscle groups and hence your body in entirety. The amount of weight used for training should be in the low range; meaning that you use weights that are comparatively light. On the other hand, the number of repetitions in a set should be more than 12. In fact, the ideal range is between 12 and 16. The rest period between sets should be very low; preferably less than half a minute.

The third objective of weight training is improvement in aesthetics. If increase in size is what you desire, then the weights you use should be moderately heavy. In fact, the weights used should be heavy enough to make the last set a hard one to complete. The rest period between the two sets should be between a minute and two, depending on the desired level of intensity. And the number of repetitions that constitute a set should be 8 to 10. Performing the various exercises within the said parameters at a lower level of intensity makes it aptly suitable for size gains. On the other hand, performing the same exercises at a higher degree of intensity will let you achieve more muscular definition and beauty.

What Happens to Your Body When You Weight Train

Now, before you run off to the gym and start lifting with gusto, first just read on to find out what exactly happens inside your body when you strength train. To know that, we need to know how our muscle fibers function.

The muscle fibers are made up of long and cylindrical looking shapes, mostly about the size of a single human hair. These are known as myofibrils and are surrounded by a gel like substance, called the sarcoplasm. Our body is composed of more than 650 types of muscle fiber groups, and they collectively help us in moving around and doing everyday work. For instance, when you bend your arm or leg or twist your waist to the side, the muscle fibers work in opposite directions, but in tandem, so as to make that particular movement possible.

There are basically two broad categories under which the muscle fibers fall into:

Slow Twitch (Type I fibers)

When you do your aerobic exercises or cardio workout, these are the fibers which come into play, when we need to convert oxygen into fuel for a long stretch of time. Slow twitch fibers are slow to respond to stress but are very resistant to fatigue.

Fast Twitch (Type II fibers)

These are quite opposite to the first type. They are super fast in responding to any stress but they also tire equally quickly. There are two types of fast twitch fibers:

- Type II A- these have a slightly better endurance quality, and come into play while running long distances or sprinting.

- Type II X- These are of major importance to weightlifters as they activate instantly when the body is placed under huge stress, say, while lifting heavy weights.

Hypertrophy

Now, most people have this misconception that weight training will somehow, magically, increase the amount of muscle fibers in the body. This is not true. All of us are born with a certain number of muscle fibers and that won't change in our lifetime. What strength training does is to increase their size, thereby contributing to increased overall muscle mass. This increase in size is called hypertrophy. There are two kinds of hypertrophy:

1.Sarcoplasmic Hypertrophy-

Remember sarcoplasm? Yeah, the gel like substance which surrounds all the muscle fibers. Concentrating on this non-contractile fluid helps you with overall size building. In such cases, the growth of the muscle and its subsequent size is attributed to the increase in sarcoplasm. Almost 30% of the muscle size is the sarcoplasm.

2.Myofibrillar Hypertrophy-

This type of growth focuses on strengthening the myofibril, which is the part of the muscle which can contract and expand. When you strength train with a goal of increasing size, you're increasing the actual size of the muscle fiber itself, and this is precisely what gives you the sculpted, dense and taut muscled look.

There's another kind of hypertrophy where the fun part lies. Called transient hypertrophy, this is where the "pump" phase of weight lifting occurs. A pump is basically a temporary increase in muscle size, which happens during strength training, almost immediately after a heavy lift. This is because of fluid accumulation in the intracellular space. So, the next time you see someone at the gym show off his rippling biceps, announcing a pump, you know he's just full of water.

Now that we have the basic biology bits out of our way, let's focus on what actually happens when you lift heavy.

When you strength train, your muscle fibers break down. After the gym, when you are eating right and getting proper rest, the body begins its repair work. In the process of rebuilding its torn muscle fibers, the body not only burns a large number of calories, it also makes the fibers stronger and bigger than before. It keeps the fibers ready for another round of stress, and the next time it happens, these fibers will come back stronger and bigger than before. So on and so forth. As you keep increasing your weights and keep the rep ranges low, between 6-8, this will aid in muscle growth. And you will get your super awesome biceps and chest and make everyone gawk at you.

Key Pointers for Effective Strength Training

Progressive Overload-
Muscle growth is possible only due to overloading the fibers with increasing amounts of weights over a period of time. If you keep the resistance steady, your muscle fibers

will quickly adapt to it and you won't register any action on the growth front. Keep increasing the resistance or weights, even if by 2.5 pounds. Load up on weights such that you are only able to lift them for 5-6 reps. If you find yourself lifting a particular weight for more than 8 times, it's time to move on to a bigger weight. Don't let your muscle fibers hit a plateau. Of course, never sacrifice your form for heavier weights. The last rep should leave you gasping for breath and your whole body should strive to complete it.

Constant progression-

Keep increasing weights constantly, even if you do it at a slow rate. Don't go by what others are doing. If your current state of strength allows you to lift 25 pounds for 5-6 reps, then this is where you should begin. If you load up the plates on your barbell to 100 pounds and begin your workout, you will have extremely poor form and might even risk serious injury to yourself. So, keep your ego out of the door and lift properly and consistently.

Stick to your goals-

What do you aim to achieve? A lean, sculpted look? A mean, menacing bodybuilder look? Increase strength? Weight loss? Design your workout according to your aims and goals and don't waste your time following workout plans which do precious little to aid you in your quest.

Train smart, not hard-

Identify which areas of your body are the weakest and train them first. For instance, if your legs are your weak area, train them first. If you start with your biceps, then

core and then come on to your legs, you will be too tired to do proper justice to the workout. Do your squats, deadlift, leg presses early on and then go on to another body part. This allows you to put the maximum intensity into the workout and the weaker areas slowly become stronger.

Momentum does not equal lifting-

Don't swing the weights to complete a movement. If you're doing bicep curls, don't dance and let your whole body aid in lifting the weights. Only your biceps should lift the weights. If you're dancing, that means the weight is too much for you to handle. Go for a lighter weight, but lift with proper form. Do not be in a hurry to lift the heaviest weights possible. You will eventually get there, through consistent overload and proper form.

Myths Regarding Weight Training

Just like diet and nutrition, there are a million myths surrounding weight training. Let's take a look at some of the more common ones.

1.Lifting weights will make women bulky-

This is probably the number one fear females have when it comes to strength training. And probably why most of them end up spending hours and hours on the treadmill or Stairmaster or give in to cardio and aerobics. Ladies, please take note: our bodies are simply not equipped with the hormones needed to turn us into a gigantic Hulk. We do not possess testosterone, the male hormone, which is responsible for the huge mass of muscle you see in the gym. Unless a female ingests COPIOUS amounts of food, plus an array of nutritional supplements and tablets, there is absolutely no way she can gain that much size. Yes, weight training will give you the coveted sculpted look, a taut and toned waist and sleek, muscular arms. It will NOT turn you into the next Arnold Schwarzzeneger. Rest assured.

2.Muscle turns to fat when you stop lifting-

Oh, wow. I'd really like to see this happen. Muscle and fat are two extremely diverse entities. Neither will muscle turn to fat, nor will the opposite ever happen, even if you stop lifting for a while. Muscle will remain the same, unless you stop exercising altogether. Then it will just atrophy, not turn into fat. On the contrary, building muscle will banish fat from the body. It's simple-build your muscles, lose the fat.

3.One muscle group per day: the best way to train-

You keep hearing about this all the time. Leg day, biceps day, back day. In fact, Monday is officially the chest day the world over. So good luck trying to find a free bench on Mondays. This is a stupid notion- to focus on different muscle groups each day, as if the body doesn't know what's happening. It's not only foolish, it wastes a lot of time and doesn't give the desired results. Instead, focus on compound movements which recruit the maximum number of muscle groups all at once, or go for circuit training or HIIT, all of which target the entire body, increase strength and resistance and are much more effective than mere isolation exercises.

4. Lifting weights are bad for my joints-

Squats, in particular, have the dubious reputation of being bad for the joints. That is why so many people skip it and mindlessly sit on a leg press or leg extension machine. If you do the exercise wrong, of course it will adversely affect your body, joints included. Poor form will cause all sorts of pain and trouble. But studies have proven that people who took up strength training despite joint pains reported that they felt fitter and their pains disappeared after a few months of training. Weight training, per se, is not bad for the body at all, but a poor form and incorrect posture most definitely is, so work on that instead of bemoaning the myth.

Now that we're all set for weight training, let us also look into another important aspect.

Compound versus Isolation Exercises

Here's a typical schedule for most gym goers-chest and triceps on Monday, back on Tuesday, biceps on Wednesday, shoulders and lats on Thursday, abs and core on Friday and legs on Saturday. People adopt this method for years and never see any gains, despite their ability to lift more. Scary looking body hulks will strut around, grunting in pain, yelling when they beat their PR and offering broscience courses for free. Compare that with the quiet guy at the back of the gym, in the squat rack, silently doing his squats and deadlift without any noise, perhaps a few pull ups and bent over rows as well. He sees rapid gains, both in his physique and strength and eventually manages to lift the heaviest weight possible without much ado.

So, what's happening here?

The quiet guy is performing compound movements. Exercises which target his entire body and utilize the maximum muscle groups. The bodybuilders mentioned earlier were doing isolation exercises, which incorporates only one particular set of muscles, like the biceps or calves. So, which is better?

The compound ones, obviously. The merits are evident at a glance- you recruit the maximum number of muscle fibers, hit a number of body parts and simultaneously engage your heart as well. In isolation exercises, only one set of muscles keep getting exercised. It takes up a lot of your time as well, because just training one body part just isn't as effective as a total body workout. Compare ten supersets of bicep curls to three brutal yet satisfying sets of deadlift or pull ups. Which one worked on your body better?

But you can also incorporate isolation exercises into your routine, just to make sure you're at the top of your game. Throw in some bicep curls, skull crushers, concentration curls, hammer curls, leg presses every now and then, but certainly don't make them the mainstay of your workout routine.

Now that we've established that compound exercises are better than isolation, let us look at five of the most important compound exercises which give you a total body workout.

The Basic techniques and tips:

In this chapter, we shall be looking at some of the key techniques and tips that you have to keep in mind while performing the various exercises. Many of these are actually the core principles of weight training that have to be adhered to in order to train the right way. In fact, if you happen to peruse various research papers and articles published in this regard, these basic concepts and techniques could be found as a common factor in all of them. Set let us take a look at them one by one.

Sufficient Warm up:

The importance of sufficient warm up is something that cannot be stressed upon enough. It is one of those things, the importance of which everyone is aware of, but still chooses to take for granted and ignore conveniently. In fact, in all gravity of the matter, warm up is the most integral part of any exercise routine.

This has got so much of significance because, if you perform any kind of weight training without warming up your muscles, you are putting your body a huge risk of injury in the form of sprains, strains, tendon and ligament damage etc. All you need to do in order to safeguard yourself from trauma and injury is to make sure that at least 10 to 15 minutes is spent every time, performing warm up routines before you begin the actual exercises. These warm up exercises can be the basic ones such as stretching your limbs repeatedly, hopping or jogging on the spot etc. In the nutshell, give your body time to acclimatize rather than jump starting it into action by pouncing on super heavy weights.

Correct form over more weight

One of the most important, if not the most important matter to be kept in mind while training with weights is to maintain correct form and function. This is often sacrificed in the quest to lift more and heavier. This problem can actually be traced to lack of clarity in terms of priority of objectives. Understand the simple fact that the objective of weight training is to increase your strength or endurance or enhance the aesthetics of your body. And it is not to earn bragging rights between your buddies as to who can lift more weights.

Always perform the exercises with proper and correct form. The weights should be lifted in a controlled fashion without any sudden and jerky movements. Similarly, establish firmly your mind that your body will gain more when you lift with perfect form than when you lift huge weights in a sloppy manner.

Get sufficient rest

When it comes to working out with weights on a regular basis, it is extremely imperative to get sufficient rest. When I say rest, it means both the rest between two consecutive sets of exercises and also the rest between two days of workouts.

Grabbing a quick break of a minute or two is necessary because it helps your muscle fibers to recover from the exhaustion that you had thrust upon them through the last set. From what you had read in the previous chapters, you can easily come to the conclusion that weight training is a completely anaerobic activity. By virtue of this, lifting weights will induce lactate build up in the muscles. When you take a short break between sets, it provides time for the body to remove the lactate thereby letting you continue your workout.

Similarly, a day of heavy weight training will cause micro tears in your muscle fibers. Most muscle groups such as biceps, triceps or pectorals (chest) require an ideal rest period of 24 hours to recover from a heavy workout. Some others such as back muscles and thighs demand even more time. Hence it would be apt for you take a day's break between two days of exercise. But this does not mean that you have to space your workouts like this forever. Experienced bodybuilders and athletes exercise on a daily basis, although different muscle groups on each day. So as you gain more experience, the rest period that your body requires will also come down. You have to especially take care of this fact if you are a beginner. And always remember one fact; your body grows during periods of rest rather than when you exercise. Also make it a point to sleep for a minimum of 6 to 8 hours a day.

Overcome the "Plateau"

Every person who has trained with weights will experience what is called the "muscle plateau". This is basically nothing but a level that you reach when your workouts may not seem to give you the desired results. You may be lifting a decent amount of weight but still you may feel that your body has hit a plateau.

There are many methods of overcoming this plateau. This is one of the key areas where a smart exercise routine is differentiated from a merely hard one. Of the most effective techniques is to use the shock principle. In this what you do is basically bring about drastic changes in your workout schedule that shocks your body into growth.

Another method is to completely change the order of specific exercises in which you go about normally on a day. For example, if you have the habit of doing the Dumbbell Curls first, then Hammer Curls and then Concentration Curls reverse the order and start from the last. The idea is to bring as much variety into your workouts as possible so that the body does not settle into a predictable and comfortable routine that hampers growth.

Listen to your inner rhythm

This is the most important tip; always listen to your inner rhythm. Every human body has its own character and nature, literally and metaphorically. Not everybody will have the same kind and nature of development. Not everyone can have the same rate of growth by doing identical exercises. What needs to be done is figure out exactly what kind of exercise your body responds to and take that path.

To a large extent, this depends on what kind of a physique the person has. There are broadly three kind of body types; Mesomorphs, Endomorphs and Ectomorphs. Mesomorphs are those individuals who generally have a broad and muscular physical nature. Their body responds to training much better than other body types. Ectomorphs are the polar opposite. They have a very narrow and slight frame that sports a lean musculature. Endomorphs are the kind that comes in between. This is the group were a majority of people fall in.

Chapter 4: Compound Exercises: The Five Smartest Methods of Gaining Strength

Here, we take a look at some incredibly powerful exercises which boost overall strength like nobody's business.

Squats-

Rightly called the King of all exercises, squats are a total body, compound movement which uses almost all the joints and muscles of your body. If just normal, bodyweight squats are so powerful, imagine what will happen if you take a loaded barbell across your shoulders and squat. The power gets magnified manifold. It uses almost every single muscle group to complete the movement. Think about it- you stand with the loaded barbell, your back is straight, your core is tight and ready, your arms grip the barbell, your shoulder blades arch to provide it with a groove, your hamstrings and glutes are ready to bear the brunt of the squat. As you descend and ascend from the squat, you maintain the tightness in your body; otherwise the movement will not take place properly. So, you see- your legs, arms, shoulders, core, back, wrists- everything is involved in this movement.

This is also a bone loading exercise, which stimulates your bones to make them denser and stronger. Such bones are healthier and less likely to break. Despite all its benefits, squats still strike fear in people's hearts as being bad for the knees and joints. But unless done badly, squats actually strengthen your glutes, hamstrings and the entire posterior chain, making them more flexible and immune to injury. Performing squats regularly has its real life applications as well, when you can lift things with ease, do your routine jobs with far more effectiveness and generally discover a more limber you.

How to Squat Properly

First, let's see how a normal bodyweight squat is done.

- Stand with your feet slightly more than shoulder width. Turn your feet out 30 degrees, if it's comfortable. It does help you squat deeper.
- Stretch your arms in front of you. Keep your back and neck straight.
- Inhale and lower yourself, as if sitting in an imaginary chair. Squat till your legs are parallel to the ground.
- Keep your breath tight and slowly ascend from the ground, without losing the tightness in your body.

Now, let's see how it's done with a loaded barbell. You need to get inside a power rack or a squat rack for this, with catchers on either side. Before any heavy lifting, first do a couple of sets with only the rod, for a warm up.

- Select an appropriate weight and stack the barbell.
- Get under the rod and position it between your shoulder blades. Slightly arch your back so that

there is a nice groove for the rod to sit. Grip it well with both the wrists. Don't lose this form for the entire set.

- Spread your legs wider than your shoulders. Drive your heels to the ground.
- Inhale and descend slowly, keeping your back and core tight.
- Squat as deep as possible, making sure your knees don't go beyond your toes. Don't worry if they do; some people's anatomy is like that.
- Don't exhale at the bottom, keep your breath inside.
- As you ascend, drive through your heels and come back up.
- Do not let your knees wobble as you ascend.

There are different kinds of squats- front, split, Bulgarian, sumo etc. However, this is the classic and most powerful technique of building a strong body. Keep these points in mind the next time you attempt to do squats.

Deadlift-

If the squat is the king of exercises, the deadlift is the unrivalled Emperor. This amazing exercise is even more powerful than the squat. Read on to know why.

Why Deadlift is So Awesome!

1.Strengthens the back-

It builds your back like no other exercise. With a strong back, life becomes easier, doesn't it? Along with pull ups, deadlift is the number one go-to exercise for a strong back.

2.Builds core stability-

Your core strength refers to the central muscles of the body- the abdominal muscles, lower back, glutes and the obliques. A firm, solid core is equally important for all other life activities, gym included. A proper deadlift targets all the core muscle groups, giving you an absolutely correct posture and slowly builds strength, over a period of time. This enables people to keep their backs straight even in daily life activities.

3.Strengthens supporting muscle groups-

The major muscles of the legs, hamstrings, waist, arms, shoulders and chest are also strengthened with a correct deadlift technique. Not to mention the heart, which is continually in a state of becoming stronger with compound movements. It forces the body to take the stress of heavy lifting and compels the muscles to grow. Take biceps, for example. Hours and hours of curls and hammer won't give you as much growth as regular, intense sessions of deadlift. By the time you are lifting really heavy in deadlift, your biceps will also have grown enviably.

4.Real life applications-

We keep lifting things every day, but we do it in a sloppy manner. Backs bent, shoulders drooping, legs at awkward angles and so on. A regular deadlift incorporated into your workout will spill over in your real life as well. You will find yourself lifting heavy objects with a subtle grace, a straight back, a proper stance and highly diminish your chances of injury.

5.True measure of strength-

There's no hullabaloo with deadlift. Only a loaded bar and your will power. There's no yells or energy drinks or spotter or a group of guys to egg you on. Just you and your barbell.

6.Fantastic cardio-

Forget about dancing to Shakira and Gaga. A truly intense session of squats and deadlift will leave you breathless and pleading for mercy. It severely taxes the cardio-respiratory system and burns an inordinate number of calories, many hours after the exercise.

All pumped up for a deadlift? Here's how you do it.

- First, as with every exercise, warm up with a rod.
- Load the barbell with an appropriate weight. You should not be able to lift it for more than 5 reps.
- When gripping the bar, turn one of the palms towards you. This alternate grip increases your holding power.
- Place feet shoulder width wide beneath the rod such that it falls in the middle line of your shoe.
- Bend down such that your back is neutral. Neither arched nor drooped.

- Hold your arms straight, gripping the rod tightly. At this stage, you're ready to lift.
- Inhale, and steadily lift the bar towards you. Think of it as pushing the earth away from you.
- Hold for a second, then slowly lower the bar to the floor.
- As you are lowering it, keep it as close to your thighs as possible, while keeping your back neutral. This will give you more range of motion.

Deadlift has its varieties and can be done with dumbbells as well. Try this classic movement and notice the changes in your body after a few weeks.

Bench Press-

The single most favourite exercise of gym goers everywhere. It's so popular, it even has an entire day dedicated to it- Monday. Ardent gymmers worldwide put on their gear, march to the gym, locate their bench and just start bench pressing like there's no tomorrow. Maximum competition can be seen while someone is attempting a bench press. And sadly, many mishaps have also made their way into the lives of gymmers who got too enthusiastic and did not request for a spotter.

What Makes the Bench Press So Darn Popular?

1. Maximum chest muscles overload-

In its ability to target the pectoral muscles, the bench press has virtually no competition. It does this by not isolating only the chest muscles. When you bench press, the triceps, biceps and shoulders also come into the picture, along with your back, core and legs.

2.Builds upper body mass-

Along with a proper lifting routine, healthy diet and regular rest, the bench press is unrivalled in building your upper body mass. Of course, there are many good isolation exercises out there solely for the chest, but bench press beats all of them hands down when it comes to adding some real bulk to your chest.

3.Increases your push strength-

Any pushing exercise involves the pectorals, shoulders, biceps and triceps. The bench press involves all of them and thus, is a superior exercise when it comes to increasing your push strength. This strength is used for other compound movements like the overhead press or push up variations.

Let's not waste any more time and get right down to business!

How to Bench Properly

First, set up the bench correctly. The bar should be at a height which allows for full range of motion. When you hold the bar and unrack it, you should be able to lift it straight up in the air with your back firmly on the bench and neck looking up.

- Load the barbell with an appropriate weight.

- Lie flat on the bench. Keep your legs firmly fixed to the ground.
- Arch your back a little, not too much. Maintain the tightness in your core during the entire set.
- Draw your shoulder blades together, like trying to squeeze them.
- Look straight up at the bar and unrack it. Imagine that you're trying to break the bar in the middle.
- Inhale and bring it all the way down to your chest, almost touching it.
- Your elbows should be at ninety degrees from your shoulders. Do not let them flare out.
- Hold your breath and drive the rod back up forcefully, without lifting your shoulders from the bench or losing the tightness in your core. This is one rep.

Regular bench pressing will definitely increase the muscle mass in your upper body and make you stronger for other compound exercises.

The Overhead Press-

Simply put, the overhead press is unrivalled when it comes to not only building a rock solid upper body and core, but also your legs, back and arms. It is a wonderful compound movement that tests your balance as well as coordination, and a single misstep can result in severe injury.

Common Mistakes Newcomers Make

Like the bench press, overhead press also relies on precise angles and lowering phases. There are certain things to be kept in mind while attempting an overhead press, which people sadly tend to forget.

1.A compound movement, not a dance-

In their zeal and enthusiasm to lift more and more, people tend to think of the barbell as a means of dancing. They load it up merrily, swing it high in the air, use their entire body to keep it there and bring it down in a rocking fashion.

2.Not adopting a proper stance-

The correct way to stand would be directly under the bar, in line with your feet, hips thrust out very slightly, feet placed shoulder width wide and your core tight. Most newbies keep one foot forward and one at the back, like a lunge movement, mistakenly believing that this stance will help them lift more weight. This will only harm their back and spine.

3.Not keeping the arms at ninety degrees-

This movement primarily requires your arms and shoulders. For this, maximum strength is possible only when they are perpendicular to your body during the lift. If they sag or move forwards or backwards, the lift becomes more difficult.

How to Do the Overhead Press Properly

- Stand directly under the bar, such that you are able to stretch your hands out completely during the lift.
- Load the bar with an appropriate weight.
- Place your feet slightly wider than shoulder width and keep your helps firmly planted on the floor.
- Unrack the bar and first bring it to chest level. Your elbows should not flare out. Keep them straight and level.
- Inhale and slowly lift the bar above your head. When you do this, you find that your head comes in between. To avoid this, slightly tilt back as you lift the bar and bring it down.
- Hold the bar for a second and bring it down.
- During the lift, keep your head straight. Look ahead. Don't look up or down towards the bar.

Barbell Rows-

Another wonderful and powerful compound exercise, barbell or bent over rows are exceptional for building your back, both upper and lower, not to mention your hamstrings, glutes and the entire posterior chain. Plus, you use your arms and core to pull and push the bar towards the ground so your entire body gets a tremendous workout.

Benefits of Barbell Rows

1.Good posture-

Continual incorporation of rows in your workout will surely give you a strong and good posture, as you develop a shapely and appealing back.

2.Everyday applications-
Just like the deadlift, barbell rows will strengthen your whole body. The next time you lift heavy furniture or bags of groceries or climb stairs with heavy water cans, you will thank this movement.

3.Builds a strong back-
With a well built back, you can perform much better in other exercises as well as in real life.

Now, let's see how this is done, all right?

How to Do the Barbell Row?

- Adopt a stance just like in deadlift. Feet shoulder width apart, bend at the waist till your back is parallel to the ground and straight, feel the stretch in your hamstrings.
- The rod should be aligned with the middle part of your foot.
- The grip changes here. Turn your palms outside and grab the rod.
- Without looking up or down, keeping the back neutral, pull the bar towards your chest, keeping it as close to the body as possible, like rowing a boat.
- Your forearms and upper back should be doing all the work.
- Hold for a second and slowly lower the bar towards the ground. This is one rep.

- Be careful not to look where the bar goes. Keep your head and eyes fixed at a particular point on the ground.
- Do not let your back come up or become rounded. If you do this, you will lose your full range of motion.

Chapter 5: Isolation Exercises

In this chapter, we shall look at what I consider to be the most effective exercises in terms of growth in strength, endurance and size. The exercises mentioned in the forthcoming pages have been picked keeping in the mind both the beginners as well as people who have been training with weights for a long time. These are all time honored techniques, which if done the right way can help you achieve what you have set out for.

You may notice that I have concentrated more on exercises that make use of free weights instead of relying on machines. That is because of the fact that, free weights stimulate your muscles better than machines in terms of growth. And this is also partly the reason why most, if not all the free weight exercises in this section make use of Dumbbells instead of Barbells. This is because of the fact that using a Dumbbell in each hand as against a Barbell, that makes use of both arms, employs all the stabilizer muscles in your arms, which go a long way in ensuring wholesome development.

I have segregated the exercises in terms of muscle groups. We will be covering the arms and shoulders first, then move on to the chest and back. Then we will look at the abdominal and at last the legs. Remember what I had mentioned in the beginning itself, the smartest way to go about weight training is to make sure that your form is correct and proper and to perform those exercises that really utilize your muscle fibers to the fullest rather than those that simply entail lifting the heaviest dumbbell in sight.

Also make it a point to adhere to the techniques and tips that I had mentioned in the previous chapter. I will not be mentioning the repetitions in each set because as I have said in detail earlier, it depends on whether you are exercising for strength or endurance or size. I will, however be mentioning the number of sets, so you can perform the desired number of repetitions as per your priority.

Arms (Biceps and Triceps)

One of the most worked on parts, biceps are a favourite amongst gym goers all around the world. True, when you want to look good in a t-shirt with short sleeves or when you want to show off your toned arms in a sleeveless top, a muscled arm is definitely on the cards. Women in particular, are mostly unhappy with the way their arms begin to sag.

The major arm muscles are the biceps brachii, the coracobrachialis, brachialis and the triceps brachii. Exercising both these sets of muscles is equally important in achieving your goal. Here are some common and easy to perform arm exercises.

Biceps

1.Squat Curls-

Seems like a weird combination, right? Well, it is and burns your legs and biceps together. Here's how you do it: squat normally till your thighs are parallel to the ground. As you descend, bring the dumbbells towards your shoulders, in a normal bicep curl. As you ascend from the squat, lower them towards the ground. That's one rep.

2.Front leaning concentration curls-

- Bend at the waist and stretch your right hand forward, in a slant. The other hand will be at the back of your waist.
- Hold the dumbbell straight down and curl the wrist a little inwards. Now move the dumbbell towards the inner side of your shoulder and keep your wrist tucked in. This gives you a nice pump in your biceps.

3.Side hammer curls-

- Cross your right hand in front of your chest such that it is parallel to your waist.
- Hold the dumbbell straight and move it down till your hand is parallel to your right leg. Without a break, bring it back up again to waist level. This is one rep.

4.Curls with weighted rods-

Chuck the dumbbells for some serious action with the barbell.

- First warm up with the rod. Add weights to it till you are comfortable with it and hold the rod with both hands, wrists facing you.
- Pull the bar to your shoulders and make sure only your biceps and forearms do all the work. Don't swing or make your back do the work.

5.Squat Cable Pull up-

Sounds funny? Do it once, it's no laughing matter.

- Stand in front of the cable machine and add a comfortable weight to it.
- Keep the cable at such a level that when you squat, you should be able to pull it towards you.
- Squat till your legs are parallel to the ground and pull the cable towards you, like a normal bicep movement. Remain in the squat position till one complete set is over. Not so easy now, is it?

6.Single hand cable-

- Add appropriate weight to the cable and keep one handle in your hand.
- Stand such that the handle in aligned with your wrist. Keep some distance from the cable so that when you pull it towards you, only your biceps perform the movement.
- Pull the handle towards you, and keep your elbows in line with your shoulder. This ensures that only

your biceps do all the work. Release the handle slowly. This is one rep.

7.Standing alternate dumbbell curls-

These are arguably the most instantly recognizable exercise in the word. And it doesn't hurt when the recognition is rivaled only by the efficacy of the exercise.

- In order to perform them, stand upright with a pair of dumbbells in your hand. Your feet should be shoulder width apart.

- Now with elbows stationary, curl the weights up alternatively, one hand at a time. Watch your breathing; inhale while the weight is lowered and exhale when lifting. Perform 4 to 6 sets.

8.Standing alternate hammer curls-

This exercise is very similar to the previous exercise.

- Stand in the same position with your arms hanging by your side, carrying dumbbells. What you have to do is change the way you hold the dumbbells.

- Grasp the weights in such a way that the palms and fingers are facing inwards towards the body. Raise and lower the weights in the same fashion as you would with a hammer. Perform 4 to 6 sets.

9.Sitting concentration curls-

- Sit down on the edge of a bench and bend over.

- Now lift a dumbbell and place your elbow firmly against the inside of your knee. Lift the weight towards your shoulder and lower it.

- Once the desired repetitions have been completed for one arm, shift you position and repeat the motion with the other arm. Inhale when lowering the weight and exhale while lifting. Perform 4 to 6 sets.

Triceps

1.Reverse rod curls-

- Grab a barbell and load it with appropriate weights.
- Hold it such that your wrists face inwards. Now pull it towards you, keeping your elbows straight, such that only the triceps bear the full brunt of the movement.

2.Cable push down-

- Adjust the weight in the machine.
- Keeping your arms and back straight, pull the lever towards the ground till your arms are straight.
- Bring it back up slowly with your elbows straight. You will feel the stretch and pull in your triceps.

3.Overhead cable push-

- Stand in such a way that the cable is behind and above you.

- Stretch your arms backward and grab the bar.
- Step a few meters away from the cable and pull the lever all the way above your head, keeping your arms straight.
- Without losing the tension in your body, gently bend your arms at the elbows and take the lever back. This is one rep. Be careful not to lose your balance.

4.Overhead tricep dips-

You can do this either sitting or standing. If sitting, keep your back straight and attached to the chair wall. If standing, keep your back straight and your legs shoulder width wide.

- Take a suitably heavy dumbbell and grab it with both hands such that your palms take the weight of the dumbbell.
- Take it all the way behind your head.
- Only bend your arms at the elbows and let the dumbbell go all the way behind your head towards the ground. When you feel a stretch in your triceps, slowly bring the dumbbell back up above your head. This is one rep.

5.Skull crushers-

Don't worry; this won't harm your skull at all.

- Lie on a flat bench with your legs firmly on the ground.
- Take a straight or curled barbell (this works better, for some reason) and stretch your hands all the way up, palms away from you.
- Now, just bend them at the elbow, keeping the rest of the forearms straight, and bring the rod as close to your forehead as possible. Lift it slowly back up till your hands are straight again.

6.Narrow grip rod push-

- Lie on a flat bench.
- Grab a barbell, palms facing away, like a normal bench press.
- This time, bring your hands really close together, creating a narrow distance between then.
- Push it up, keeping your hands straight and lower them towards your chest. This creates tension in your triceps.

7.Parallel bar dips-

- Stand in the middle of a standard set of parallel bars and prop yourself up using the arms.

- Now lower the body until the arms are bent at 90 degrees at the elbow.

- Hold this position for a moment and push yourself up again till the elbows are a little short of locking

out. Inhale when lowering the weight and exhale while lifting. Perform 4 to 6 sets.

8.Dumbbell kickbacks-

- Pick up a dumbbell and bent over halfway with your back straight.

- Bring the arm with the weight in line with your torso while holding on to the edge of a bench for support with the other arm.

- Now push the arm with the weight back, as much as it can go without moving the elbow. Inhale when lowering the weight and exhale while pushing the weighted arm back. Perform 4 to 6 sets and the repeat with the other arm.

Shoulders

With a drool worthy chest, it's time to work the shoulders. In order to get well sculpted shoulders, you need to hit all the muscles which make them up. These are the deltoids, the rotator cuff, trapezius, serratus anterior, subclavius and pectoralis minor.

Given below are some bodyweight shoulder exercises, ranging from easy to hard. Take it easy and do not jump headfirst into the hardest exercise first. If unsuccessful, you might give it up altogether. You might dismiss off the shoulder exercises as being too mundane, but possessing strong shoulders give also give you overall strength.

In order to pack some muscle into your shoulders, keep the rep range low, between 6-10, and also increase the time under tension. Try the following exercises carefully and with proper form.

1. Single Arm Plank-

- Get down on all fours. Straighten your legs and your core.

- Lower your hands till your elbows form a ninety degree angle with your shoulders. Keep them beneath your shoulders. This is your standard plank position.

- Now, extend your right hand forward, as if reaching for something, keeping the rest of your body in a straight line. Hold for a few seconds.

- Let the hand back in its original position and extend the left hand forward.

2. Crab walk-

This is a great exercise for shoulder strength, which uses the stabilizer muscles and the deltoids. Try walking backwards, if you need a challenge!

- Sit with your hands behind your shoulders.

- Slowly lift your hips, letting your glutes hang in the air, with your knees bent.

- Walk forward, with your right leg and left arm, then your left leg and right arm.

- Brace your shoulders and keep them tight. Repeat as many rounds as you can.

3. Planche Push up-

This is an awesome gymnastics skill exercise in which the body is held parallel to the ground, supported by the arms and shoulders. It requires great strength and balance. To make it slightly easier, a push up version of the planche is given below.

- Get down on the floor, in a normal push up position.

- Instead of placing your hands directly below your shoulders, make a ninety degree angle with your waist. Your palms should be at the sides of your waist, the elbows in a straight line with your back. Think of the chaturanga pose in Yoga.

- Keeping the body straight, lift yourself up, hold for a few seconds, then lower the body till it is parallel to the floor. This is one rep. Do as many as possible without losing form.

4. Elevated Pike push up-

- Get into a normal push up position.

- Keep your feet on an elevated surface, such as a table or a bed or a bench.

- Bend your hips, raising your hips and butt towards the ceiling, such that your torso is vertical.

- Lower yourself to the floor until your head is between your hands. Get back up explosively.

5.Military press-

This is the most common version of the exercise and be done in a sitting or standing position. In both positions, keep your back straight.

- Hold the dumbbells in your hands such that your palms are facing out.

- Raise your arms above your head and stretch them, bringing the dumbbells close together in the air. Hold for a second.

- Bring them back to shoulder level. This constitutes one rep.

6.Arnold press-

This is somewhat similar to the military press, but the direction of the hands changes mid air.

- Hold the dumbbells in line with your shoulders.

- As you raise your arms, rotate your wrists such that the dumbbells face each other mid air.

- When you bring your hands down, rotate them back in the original position.

7.Single hand press-

In this variation, you do the military press one hand at a time.

- Hold the dumbbells aligned with the shoulders.

- Lift your right hand high above your head, exhale and bring it back down, simultaneously lifting your left hand above your head.

8.Dumbbell Overhead Presses-
- Sit on the edge of a bench and take two moderately heavy dumbbells in your hand.

- Maintain the torso erect and bend your arms at the elbows completely so that the dumbbells are resting at shoulder height. This is the starting position.

- Now push the weights up in a straight line and hold for a moment before lowering the weights. Inhale when lowering the weight and exhale while pressing the weights up. Perform 4 to 6 sets.

9.Dumbbell Lateral Raises-

- Pick up a pair of low weight dumbbells and stand with your feet shoulder width apart.

- Hold the weights by your sides, palms facing inwards.

- Slightly bent your elbows and raise the weights up to the sides, hold for a moment and bring it down.

- Make sure the weights do not go higher than shoulder level when raised. Inhale when lowering the weight and exhale while lifting. Perform 4 to 6 sets.

10.Dumbbells Front Raises-

- Adopt the same starting position as the above exercise with nearly the same weights, except with a slight alteration.

- Keep the arms in front, weights hanging in front of the thighs.

- Now raise them to the front, not above the shoulder level. This variation hits the front shoulder muscles. Inhale when lowering the weight and exhale while lifting. Perform 4 to 6 sets.

Chest

Your chest is made up of four major muscle groups, namely, the pectoralis major, the pectoralis minor, subclavius and the serratus anterior. In order to get the optimum results, all of these muscle groups need to be worked on. While weight training, one has the advantage of progressively overloading the muscles every week or with each set. With bodyweight training, however, the key focus should be on the time each muscle group is kept under tension. Since the muscle fibers cannot be overloaded week after week, the time under tension will provide the resistance necessary to build the muscle. The human body does not know whether the resistance is from a barbell or a dumbbell or a cable or its own weight. All it knows is that something is pushing it or it has to pull something. Of course, as with every exercise, proper form is of utmost importance. You need to hit the full range of motion in every single rep. Cheating and poor form will get you nowhere.

All right, now that we have the basics out of the way, let's get started on the exercises. Aim to get at least 5-7 reps on each set. It will get better as you get stronger.

1.Dumbbell bench press-

Tired of the same old barbell? Try this, and you'll wonder about the range and the depth.

- Take two dumbbells of appropriate weight and lie on a flat bench.
- As with the normal bench press set up, arch your back a little, keep your hands straight and legs firmly on the ground.
- Inhale and lower your arms till the dumbbells are parallel to your shoulders. Straighten your arms again. This is one rep. The reason why you feel a

better pump with this exercise is because dumbbells allow for a greater range of motion and increased depth.

2.Incline and decline bench press-

This can be done with either dumbbells or a barbell. When doing an incline press, make sure you can straighten your arms to their fullest without getting your back off the bench. When doing decline press, first balance your body on the bench properly, else you risk severe injury. The decline press allows the maximum range of motion possible.

3.Dumbbell flies-

- Lie on a flat bench and keep two dumbbells in your hands.
- Straighten your arms such that the dumbbells face each other.
- Arch your back a little. Now pull your hands down in the opposite direction till each hand is parallel to the ground on its side. Right hand swings in the right direction, the left hand goes in the left direction.
- Without looking up or straining your neck, slowly bring your hands together.

4.Reverse flies-

- Lay down on your stomach on the bench or an incline bench.

- Your hands should be straight down, holding the dumbbells.
- Keep your head neutral and slowly lift your arms till they are parallel to the floor. Slowly bring them back to their original position. This is one rep.

5.The Butterfly-

- As with the one arm bicep pulley curl, stand in such a way that each of the arms is aligned with the handle of the pulley.
- Keep one leg in the front for support and pull both the handles towards the ground, keeping your arms straight and chest out.
- Without losing momentum, slowly bring your arms to their sides again.

6.Push Up and its Variations-

Simply put, the push up is one of the best exercises not just for the chest, but the core and arms as well. In a regular push up, one gets into the push up position on all fours, back straight, arms just below the shoulders, and lowers the body to the ground in a straight line until the chin almost touches the floor and then back up. Let's look at some variations of the push up:

a. Incline Push up-

People who have trouble doing the basic push up can start with this. This exercise targets the main chest muscles but puts less pressure on the elbows and also considerably reduces the amount of body weight which is being lifted. Incline push ups can be done against any solid surface, such as a desk, a wall, a table top etc.

- Face the surface (table or a desk or a wall) and place your arms, a bit wider than you shoulder width.

- With your body in a straight line, bend forward until your face is close to the surface of the wall or table. Make sure your back is rigid all this time. Go back to the starting position.

b. Decline Push up-

This is slightly harder in intensity than an incline push up. Your feet are elevated and you need to exert more force in your arms to lift your body to maintain the level.

- Choose an elevated surface, like a chair or a bed or a bench. Make sure the height of the chosen surface is not more than you can handle.

- Place your feet on the surface, your hands below your shoulder line and the entire body in one straight line.

- Lower your body such that your hands are perpendicular to your shoulders. Do not let your hips sag or your back bend. Quickly, lift your body to its earlier position.

c. Wide Hand Push up-

The hands are placed slightly wider apart than with a normal push up hand width. The movement is the same, and this variation targets your biceps as well as your pecs.

d. Diamond Push up-

Nothing beats this exercise when it comes to sculpting a great looking chest. Plus, it targets your triceps as well.

- Get in the push up position. Form a diamond with your hands and place them beneath your shoulders.

- Keeping your abs, glutes and back tight and straight, lower yourself to the floor and keep your elbows close to your body.

- Lift yourself up the same way.

e. Cross Over Box Push up-

This one is great for building your strength as well as your chest. You need an object like a sturdy box or a plate which can be fixed at one point.

- Adopt a push up position, with one hand on the box or plate.

- Lower yourself and while lifting your body switch your hands explosively, so that the other one lands on the object. That's one rep.

- Alternate hands while lifting yourself up.

f. Spiderman Push up-

- Get into a normal push up position.

- As you lower your body, bring your right knee up to your right elbow. Keep it like this till you lift yourself up.

- On the next rep, bring your left leg to your left elbow. Continue for as many reps as you can do without losing form.

g. The Hindu Push up-

- Get into the push up position.

- Raise your hips high.

- When lowering yourself, instead of going in a straight line, arch your back and dive slightly, with your head and hips sticking out.

- Lower yourself until your chest reaches the ground, then lower your hips and hold the position for a few seconds. Repeat.

Back

All the time, we see gym goers focus mostly on their biceps, abs and chest. A lot of people who exercise at home also concentrate on legs, abs and arms. The back is one of the most neglected body parts, when it should occupy the first place. Why, you ask? Read on.

Why You Should Work on Your Back

✓ The back contains some of the biggest and strongest muscles in the body, only second to legs. The main muscles of the back are the trapezius, lattisimus dorsi, levator scapulae and the rhomboids. If you work on your back muscles, you will surely gain a lot of strength and power.

✓ Secondly, a chiseled, wide back also creates the illusion of a trimmer abdomen.

✓ Since most of the back exercises are compound movement, involving multiple joints and muscle groups, you will certainly burn more calories per exercise.

✓ A stronger back will aid in many other exercises, like squats, deadlift, clean and press, barbell rows etc.

Some of the best exercises for building a strong back can be divided into three categories- muscular endurance, strength, building muscle mass. Let's look at each of them separately.

Muscular Endurance

This basically means the ability of the muscle fibers to withstand the pressure and resistance of the exercise over a long period of time or a large number of reps per set.

1. Horizontal/Vertical Pull up-

Instead of a normal pull up, a beginner can start with either the horizontal or vertical pull-ups.

- To do a horizontal pull up or inverted row, get under a bar or a sturdy table.

- Grab the bar with both hands, palms facing away from you. Keeping your body in a straight line, pull yourself up till your chin reaches the bar. Lower your body in a line.

- For a vertical version, you may use door handles or a towel wrapped around a vertical structure. Grab the ends of the towel or handles. Keep your body straight and pull yourself towards the door. Get back into position without letting your back hunch.

2. Squat Pull up-

- You will need a bar for this.

- Squat on the floor, making sure your knees are in line with your toes.

- When you get back up, immediately grab the bar and pull yourself up. This is one rep.

Strength

For developing strength, your exercises should be in the 6-8-rep range.

1. One Arm Pull up-

The name itself strikes fear amongst even the elite gymmers. Mastering pull-ups will get easier with time, but one arm pulls ups are surely a test of your arm and back strength.

- Get in a basic pull up position, arms hanging straight from the bar.

- Bring one hand down to your side and use only one hand to pull yourself up completely.

2. Tuck Front Lever pull up-

The front lever is one of the toughest exercises for building a strong back. It is a gymnastic move, and most people are not able to do even the back lever, a relatively easier version, even after months of practice. A simpler variation of this is the tuck front lever.

- Grasp the bar with an overhand grip.

- Lean back and pull your legs and hips up, forming a curve with your lower body. Your back should be rounded and the legs and knees tucked as tightly as possible.

- Now, try to pull yourself up slowly. Get back to the original position.

Building Muscle Mass

1. The Pull up-

This old time favorite is still a hot commodity as far as building back mass goes. It is definitely one of the best exercises for a wide back and shapely lats.

- Grab hold of a bar and hang all the way down. Your arms should be straight. The grip should be slightly wider than your shoulders.

- Pull yourself up until your chin is above the bar. Your back may form a slant at this point, but that's all right.

- Lower yourself all the way down.

- Do not swing your body for the momentum. All the work has to be done by your arms and back muscles.

2. Isometric Pull up Holds-

This is done in three phases.

- Pull yourself up in a normal pull up position and hold it for 30-45 seconds.

- Lower yourself down, hanging straight, and rest for 30 seconds. Then pull yourself up such that your elbows are bent at 90 degrees. Hold for 15 seconds. Lower yourself and rest for 30 seconds.

- From a dead hang, pull yourself up only 2 inches and hold for 15-20 seconds. This constitutes one rep.

Abs and Core

The abdominal muscles or abs are perhaps the most worked on body part everywhere. Whether it is a gym or within the comfort of one's home, people everywhere are obsessed with getting a flat, toned tummy. While the male population hankers after the six packs, the females are preoccupied about getting a bikini ready body.

Normally, in order for the abs to show, the body fat levels in a male should be at 6-8%, while a female should be at 12-13%. When the core muscles become stronger and show definition, it will burn the abdominal fat. Plus, a proper diet goes a long way in giving you results.

Forget about torturing your abs with hundreds of crunches and sit-ups. They do not make any difference to banish the fat around your midsection. Instead, try the following exercises to strengthen your core and get those muscles to pop out.

1. The Plank-

This one isometric exercise truly blasts and destroys your abs. It strengthens the whole body, build a strong core, strengthen the back and also build your shoulders.

- Get into a push up position.

- Bend your elbows 90 degrees and rest your weight on your forearms. They should be directly under your shoulders.

- Form a straight line with your body and hold on to this position as long as you can. Do not let your hips sag.

2. Side Crunch-

Along with the core, it also works the obliques.

- Kneel on the floor, place your right palm on the floor and lean towards your right side.

- Balance your weight, slowly extend your left leg and point your toes ahead.

- Place your left hand behind the head, making sure the elbow points towards the ceiling.

- Lift your leg to your hip height as you extend your arm above your leg, palm facing forward. Lower to the starting position.

3. Opposite Arm and Leg Raise-

- Get down on all fours.

- Slowly, extend your right leg behind to hip height, in line with your back.

- At the same time, extend the left hand forward. Hold for a few seconds.

- Go back to the original position. Alternate the hand and the leg.

4. Single Leg Stretch-

- Lie on your back, with your knees bent.

- As you inhale, pull in your left knee towards your chin, while raising your head to meet it.

- Lift your right leg about 45 degrees from the floor.

- Switch legs. Hold the position for at least 10 seconds.

5. Side Plank with Leg Lift-

- Get into a basic side plank position.

- Press your bottom foot firmly on the ground and raise the top leg as high as you can, without dropping your hips.

6. Flutter Kicks-

This is a fantastic exercise for your hip flexors as well as your abdominal muscles.

- Lie on your back with your arms at your sides.

- Extend your legs in the air, keeping them slightly bent at the knees.

- Lift your heels about 5 inches off the floor and make small, rapid scissor like movements. Keep your abs contracted all this time.

7. Russian Twist-

Another wonderful exercise that targets the abs and obliques at once is the Russian Twist

- Sit on the ground with your knees bent. Keep your heels close to your butt.

- Lean back slightly, keeping the back straight.

- Extend your hands in the front and twist slowly to the left. Don't swing. Let the ribs and the abdominal muscles do the work. Twist to the right side. This is one rep.

8.Crunches-
- Lie down on your back and keep the arms tied behind the back.

- Bend your knees at around 45 degrees, feet flat on the floor.

- Now raise your torso while crunching your stomach. The aim is to perform the crunching action perfectly, instead of simply sitting up. Inhale when lowering the torso and exhale while crunching. Perform 4 to 6 sets

9.Leg Raises-

- Lie down on the bench on your back.

- Now keep legs straight, the toes close to each other
  and raise them together, about 45 degrees off the
  level of your torso.

- Hold the position for a moment and bring the legs
  down slowly. Make sure that the actions are done
  deliberately and not in a jerking fashion. Inhale
  when lowering the legs and exhale while lifting.
  Perform 4 to 6 sets.

Legs

The main muscles of the legs are quadriceps, hamstrings,
adductors (thighs); tibialis anteriors (shins),
gastrocnemius and soleus muscles make up the calves. The
legs support the entire body weight and therefore must be
exercised regularly. The following exercises are compound
movements that will work almost all the muscle groups in
the leg.

1.Leg press-

There are two kinds of leg presses. One, where you sit and
push the weight away from you and the other, where your
back is on the floor and you almost lie prone, pushing the
weight away from you. Pick any of the methods but be
extremely careful about bending your legs in the right
manner, else you risk a severe back and spine injury.

Exercise

- Get in front of the leg press machine and adjust the weight. If you're lying prone, you need to add the weight plates.

- Bend your knees till they reach your chest.

- Slowly, straighten them out again but make sure not to keep the legs stiff. Keep them bent slightly at the knees. This is one rep.

2.Leg extension-

This works well to strengthen the knee flexors and hamstrings.

- Select an appropriate weight on the machine.
- Keep your legs firmly fixed under the padded bar.
- Without momentum or explosive activity, slowly raise both your legs until they are parallel to the floor. Hold for two seconds. Lower them gently.

3.Walking lunges with weights-

A brilliant exercise that opens up your hip flexors, activates your glutes and gives you core stability.

- Extend one leg in front and keep the other leg straight. Balance the dumbbells or barbell properly in your hands or across your shoulders.

- Bend till the knee of the forward leg is perpendicular to the floor.

- Keep your back straight and don't let the knee fall over the toe line.

- As you rise, bring the back leg in the front and bend down. Keep alternating the legs as you walk. Don't let your back sag or lose its tightness.

4.Squat Jumps-

A fantastic pylometric exercise that not only works the legs but gets your heart rate bursting as well.

- Get into a deep squat position.

- When you come up, jump as high as you can and slowly land on your knees.

- Go back into the squat position.

5.Bulgarian Split Squats-

- Place one leg on a chair or a bench and extend the other leg in front of you as far as you can without losing balance.

- Bend down, keeping the knee at a 90-degree angle and the back straight. Come back up. This is one rep.

6.Deep Side Lunges-

A deeply underestimated exercise, this works wonderfully to strengthen the legs.

- Stand with your feet shoulder wide apart.

- Bend towards your right, push your hips lower and lower your body by pushing the right knee at a 90-degree angle.

- Keep the heels firmly planted on the floor and stretch as much as you can. Return to the starting position.

6.Lunge Kicks-

- Get into a basic lunge position.

- As you rise, bring your back leg to the front and explosively kick as high as you can.

- Take it to the back again and lower your body. This is one rep.

7.Glute Kicks-

- Get down on all fours.

- Keeping your back and arms straight, bring the right knee up to your chest.

- Take the whole leg back and stretch it behind you, as high as you can go.

- Bring it back to your chest. This is one rep.

8.Overhead squats-

Regular squats not your style. How about this more complex and taxing version?

Take a barbell (add weights as you become more comfortable) and hold it high up in the air, keeping your arms straight. Holding this position, squat down till your thighs are parallel to the floor. Hold for a second. Slowly ascend from the squat but don't let the bar down. This is one rep.

9.Front squats-

Load the barbell with appropriate weights. Instead of placing it between the shoulder blades, place it the front of your shoulders, near the clavicle. Hold the bar such that your palms are turned out and you find a comfortable groove between both the shoulder blades. Keeping your back neutral, slowly descend to the floor until your legs are parallel to the ground. Then, gently come up without giving any jerky movements.

10.Sumo squats-

You can do this using dumbbells or a barbell. The only thing different here is the stance. Adopt a wider-than-shoulder-level stance and squat till the thighs are parallel to the floor and the knees do not go beyond your toes. Hold for a second and return to your original position.

11.Calf Raises-

- Stand at the edge of the base of a tall machine, heels of your feet hanging out and heavy weights in hand.

- Now raise your body as much as you can, using the power of your calf muscles alone. Inhale when lowering coming down and exhale while stretching up. Perform 4 to 6 sets of 15 to 20 repetitions.

Now that we've covered the basics of the compound and isolated exercises, it's time to turn our attention to some other forms of exercise which will induce weight loss, fat loss, increased metabolism and overall strength.

Chapter 6: HIIT - A Smarter Way to Lose Weight

HIIT, or high-intensity interval training, or Tabata training is a technique in which one goes does an exercise for a given period of time in its full intensity, then takes a micro break of a few seconds before continuing the next set. It is basically a series of quick, intense bursts of exercise, with very short recovery periods. The greatest advantage with this technique is that your heart rate speeds up in no time and you also burn more fat in a less amount of time. You may feel your muscles begin to strain and feel like they're on fire. This is nothing but Excess Post-exercise Oxygen Consumption (EPOC). During the EPOC stage, the anaerobic system takes over. While exercising, the phosphate in the blood is used up first, and then lactic acid and glycolysis come into play, giving you the "burn" in your muscles. Any sort of intense exercise definitely gets your metabolism running in high gear, help you burn more fat. Some benefits of HIIT are:

1. It increases your rate of metabolism. That means, your body will continue burning calories long after you've stopped exercising, in order to replenish all the lost oxygen. This after burn effect continues up to 48 hours of your workout. You might just be sitting still, but you'll still burn calories.

2. Less time is wasted with HIIT workouts. Hardly 20-25 minutes is what is required. These workouts can be done anywhere, anytime. If you're hard pressed for time, or have only 20-30 minutes every alternate day, this is perfect for you.

3. It does not require the use of any equipment like dumbbells or barbells or kettle bells. HIIT mainly uses the bodyweight and focuses primarily on getting the heart rate up and optimum muscle building. You may also make use of weights if you feel that bodyweight is not enough for you. But as is the case with any weight training, make sure your form is absolutely proper else you might risk severe injury to your body.

Such intense burst of activity stimulates the muscle building hormones, such as the growth hormone and the IGF-1. Intense circuits stimulate your muscle-building hormones such as the growth hormone or IGF-1. This, in turn, prepares your body to shed its fat and build lean muscle mass. The shorter resting time between sets ensures that your cardiovascular health is also improved, making you recover faster from sets in future workouts.

HIIT places a lot of stress on your body. It needs time to heal after the workout, so do not do HII T more than 3 times a week. On alternate days or rest days, you may do some light cardio or strength training, but also make sure that you keep one day completely off from any sort of training. As I said before, muscles are built not while exercising, but while resting.

All right then, gear up! Get ready to blast your body through an amazing workout which will have far greater returns than you can imagine now. Perform each exercise for 20 seconds, going all out. Then rest for 10 seconds. Exercise for 20 seconds, rest 10 seconds. Complete 8 rounds of each exercise. Rest for 1 minute before going on to the next one.

A Basic HIIT workout:

Warm up- static or dynamic. Although, a dynamic warm up is better. Jog in place for 30 seconds, 30 Jumping Jacks and 30 seconds jump rope.

- Squats (with or without weights)

- Push ups

- Sit ups

- Jump squats

- Tricep dips

- Pull ups

- 30 second burpees

For sit ups, lie down on your back, with your knees bent. Keeping your core tight, raise your head and back off the ground, towards your chest, until your back is at a 90 degree angle to the floor. Hold for a few seconds and get back to the starting position.

For burpees, get into a squat position. Squat till your hips are almost parallel to the ground. Bring your hands in the front and explosively jump back, straightening your legs behind you, in a push up position. Jump back in, to a squat, and as you rise, jump as high as possible. Return to the squat position.

If this becomes too easy for you, try the other two workouts given below. You may also do them as a circuit. Do not rest in between sets while doing a circuit. Do as many reps as possible within 20-25 seconds.

Workout 1 –

Round One- burpees, mountain climbers, Jumping Jacks, jump rope for 3 minutes

Round Two- walking lunges, reverse lunges, squats, pull ups, plank, jump rope for 3 minutes.

In reverse lunges, instead of bringing the leg in the front, bring the leading leg behind and keep the alternate leg straight.

Round Three- burpees, squats, skater's lunges, diver's push ups, jump rope for 3 minutes.

For skater's lunges, stand with your feet slightly wider than shoulder width. Bring your right foot behind the left one, as far as it can go and bend both knees into a lunge. Keep the right foot behind the left heel. Return to the starting position and change the legs.

For diver's push ups, make an inverted "V" shape with your body, your hands straight, your legs stretched out behind and your hips in the air. Lower your body until your chest is almost parallel to the ground, then raise your body upwards, like a cobra. At this point, your chest should be out, your back arched, arms straight. Hold it and return to the starting position.

A slightly advanced HIIT routine is given below. Do the exercises in pairs, A and B. Do each one for 20-25 seconds, as many reps as possible, then rest for 10 seconds. Continue till you complete 8 rounds of each pair.

Workout 2-

A-Star jumps

B- Clapping push ups

For star jumps, get into a squat position. As you rise, jump up explosively, but this time, extend your hands and legs as you jump, so that your body resembles the shape of a star. Land lightly on your knees and resume the squat position.

In clapping push ups, as you lift your body up from the floor, bring both your hands together very quickly and place them back in position as you get ready for lowering yourself down.

A-Squat jumps

B- Crunches

A-Jumping lunges

B-Back bow crossovers

For the crossovers, lie on your stomach. Slowly, extend your hands in front of you as if reaching for something. Simultaneously, lift your legs from the ground as high as they can go, so that your whole body is supported on your stomach.

A- Double burpees

B- B-Hindu push up

For double burpees, stand with your feet hip wide apart, squat down and place your hands in front of your body. Kick back explosively and do two push ups. Come back to the starting position, do two back lunges and stand again. This is one rep.

Plank - for 60 seconds

Chapter 7: CrossFit Training

According to the definition given on the official site, "CrossFit is the principal strength and conditioning program for many police academies and tactical operations teams, military special operations units, champion martial artists and hundreds of other elite and professional athletes worldwide"

If you want it in simple terms, CrossFit is a program which provides you with a set of extremely challenging and varied workouts, which boost your strength and stamina. Every day, there is a new workout, called Workout of the Day (WOD). It will test a different aspect of your functional strength. CrossFit tests the entire body's strength, not just one particular set of muscles. A CrossFit training program ensures that your body is prepared for virtually anything.

It is unlike any gym you've been to before. It's not a commercial gym per se. There are no elliptical machines, Stairmasters, weight machines or Zumba or aerobics. What's so different about it? Well, read on.

Who Should Do CrossFit?

The official says that the program "is designed for universal scalability making it the perfect application for any committed individual regardless of experience."

What this means is the only requirement to join a CrossFit program is tenacity, dedication, resolve and commitment. Age, gender, flexibility no bar. You'll learn it eventually.

Each day, there is a workout posted in the site. It is not custom designed for each individual. Rather, each person does the workout to the best of his or her ability. For example, if the workout specifies squats with 140 pounds on the barbell, and if you're only able to do it with the bar (45 pounds), that is your starting point. Never mind the guy next to you who is doing squats at 200 pounds per set. If 45 pounds is what you can do right now, that's where you'll start. Also, there are provisions for exercise substitutions. If you are unable to do squats or pull ups or lunges, a similar movement will be substituted according to your ability and flexibility. Eventually, as you get stronger, you will be able to do the workouts as prescribed on the site or given by the instructor.

Why CrossFit?

1. It's a great place to start your weight training in a non judgmental and supportive environment. No one cares if you can't lift 100 pounds on a deadlift. If you can just lift the rod with proper form, you're good to go. People who are scared to try out weights at a regular gym or those who feel conscious of others watching and judging them as they do so will be able to build confidence in a CrossFit environment.

2. Some people need more encouragement and community support and ambience to start their workouts. Well, CrossFit's the ideal place for that. It has a tight knit feeling to it. Members don't just pop in to show their biceps off or grunt and yell their way towards a PR of a 500 pound deadlift. They will support and care for the newbies and heartily encourage anyone who needs help.

3. Are you someone who loves to workout every single day and feel like you've lost a loved one when you don't? Well, you'll get addicted to CrossFit in no time. Though the program is structured to give a day off in between, CrossFit fanatics end up in the gym every day, some even come in twice a day.

Is CrossFit Dangerous? Will I Hurt Myself?

There have been a lot of concerns and apprehensions regarding a CrossFit program. Let's check out a few facts about it.

1. In a typical CrossFit workout, there is a target to be met. You need to complete a certain number of exercises, be it strength training or bodyweight or cardio as fast as possible in a certain amount of time. This is where your form can go for a toss. You might be in a hurry to complete the workout within the time limit and sacrifice form for reps. Therefore; you need an experienced and certified trainer who can keep an eye on your form. This is essential as you progress onto heavy lifting with speed. If done incorrectly, it is

the fastest way of injuring yourself and you might end up with severe injuries in the long term.

2. Some of the CrossFit members do end up with a rather incredibly serious medical condition known as rhabdomyolysis. It is very rare. This occurs when people push themselves too hard all of a sudden. The muscle fibers break down and enter the kidneys, poisoning them. This condition is mostly found in ex-athletes or weightlifters that haven't exercised for a while, who return to the gym to prove to the others how much they can lift, regardless of what their body is telling them.

So yes, if you try to do something too fast and too much, it will inevitably cause a strain on your body. Go slow and go steady.

Your First CrossFit Class- What to Expect?

So, you've signed up for your first ever CrossFit class. Here's what will happen:

1. A Dynamic warm up-

This does not mean simply running on the treadmill for ten minutes. This includes movements like Jumping Jacks, jump rope, burpees, squats, push-ups, pull ups etc. These type of functional movements will complement the workout you will be doing.

2. Skill/strength work-

If it is a strength day, you will work on compound lifts like squats, deadlift, bench press, and barbell rows. If it is a skill day, you will focus on strengthening muscle groups, with exercises like pistol squats or one-hand push-ups.

3. WOD-

The workout of the day is posted on the site or given by the instructor. You need to complete a set of exercises within a limited time period. You can do that according to your level of fitness.

4. Cool down-

A series of stretches and cooling down movements, which will balance out the rigorous activity your body, has just endured. Do not skip this step.

Example of a workout:

5 pull-ups, 10 push ups, 15 squats, 20 lunges at 20 minute AMRAP (as many rounds as possible in 20 minutes)

You set your times for 20 minutes and do a circuit of the exercises, without any break between the sets. As soon as you finish your lunges, go back to the pull-ups and over and over again till the time limit is over.

CrossFit for Beginners

Intimidated by the regime? Wondering how and where to start? Here are some pointers for you:

This regime is based on ten crucial and principal physical qualities- cardio, endurance, stamina, strength, power, agility, flexibility, accuracy, coordination and balance. There are different exercises that test each of the qualities and you will do them either in pairs or groups or as a whole workout. At the end of the regime, your body should be fit enough to endure anything. The exercises are grouped together as follows:

Aerobic activity (cardio, stamina, endurance)- running, jogging, walking, swimming, jumping rope

Gymnastics (flexibility, strength, coordination, balance)- Handstands, rope climbing, trampoline exercises, ring exercises

Calisthenics (coordination, flexibility, strength)- functional movements like squats, lunges, sit ups, pull ups, push ups, crunches

Pylometrics (power and speed)- jumps, squat jumps, burpees

Weight lifting- snatch, clean and jerk

Powerlifting- squats, deadlift, bench press

Bodyweight- any functional exercise

Here are some workouts to get you started. If you can do the beginner level easily, you may move on to the advanced level.

Beginner CrossFit Bodyweight Workout-

Workout 1- 10 minutes, AMRAP

5 pull-ups, 10 push ups, 15 squats

Workout 2- Three rounds; 21,15,9 reps

Burpees, reverse lunges, pull ups

Workout 3- Three rounds, 3 minutes, 2 minute rest between rounds, AMRAP

15 sit ups, 15 walking lunges, 15 push-ups

Advanced CrossFit Bodyweight Workout-

Workout 1- 15 minutes, AMRAP

One legged squats, pull ups, dips

Workout 2- three rounds, 3 minutes, 1 minute rest between rounds

Exercise

Squat jumps, skater's lunges, chin-ups, push-ups

Workout 3- Three rounds; 21,15,9 reps.

Walking lunges, pull ups, burpees, side lunges

Chapter 8: Diet and Nutrition

Ah, your favorite chapter, isn't it? Everywhere you look, in the papers, on the net, on TV advertisements, each day brings forth a new diet plan guaranteed to make your fat disappear and give you a gleaming six pack abs, all by summer. There are so many myths surrounding this particular aspect of health, it's staggering. A perennially popular topic for discussion worldwide, nothing bonds people like an intense debate on weight loss tips and techniques.

People everywhere are desperate to lose weight and keep following fads and diets and yet fail miserably in their quest. So, what exactly is weight loss? It refers to an overall reduction in body mass, be it loss of adipose tissue, water, lean mass, connective tissue or fluids in the body. This can either occur intentionally, through a rigorous weight loss regime, exercise, gymming, diets or unintentionally, usually signifying a serious medical condition.

People who undergo diets and extreme fads further endanger themselves on account of inadequate and insufficient nutrition. The body has lowered defenses against disease, hormonal changes, and fluctuating metabolism and invites a host of parasites and other pathogens for invasion. Unhealthy means of weight loss have always proven to be detrimental in the long run. If you do want to lose weight, do it so gradually and in a healthy manner, with adequate amounts of exercise and a proper diet.

Of course, some people, especially those suffering from weight related problems like obesity, diabetes, back problems etc. need a specific weight loss plan, but that should be done by a licensed nutritionist and fitness trainer. Any intentional weight loss has to be done systematically; otherwise it might induce lasting damage to the body.

A diet is basically a planned proportion of food groups, which is eaten at periodical intervals of the day. But in order to lose weight fast, say, by the weekend, people go on crash diets and adopt all kinds of fad diets, like eating cotton balls soaked in fruit juice or the juice-only diet or the raw salad diet or the Paleo diet. Every day, some new diet appears in the market, endorsed by so-and-so celebrity, and people just blindly follow them, without thinking about the repercussions for a second. A proper diet should include all the major food groups and the number of calories ingested depends on person to person. For instance, a 110-pound man will have a daily caloric intake of about 1550 calories. This is vastly different from the 180-pound wrestler who needs a special diet and who wants to bulk up. Though the caloric intake differs from person to person, the food being eaten should not skip any of the five major groups- carbohydrates, fats, vitamins, minerals, and protein.

There are millions of myths floating around the topics of diet and nutrition. Here are a few of them. I'm sure you've come across them at some point or the other in your life.

-Chocolate gives you acne.

-Eating after 7 pm makes you fat.

-The healthiest diet to follow is low-fat, low carb, high protein with lots of grains.

-Eat several small meals a day, instead of three large meals.

-Avoid eating egg yolks.

-Eating fat makes you fat.

-Refrain from eating dairy products, as they are full of fat and unwanted calories.

-Sugar causes diabetes.

-Brown rice is superior to white rice. Actually, don't eat rice. Carbs will make you fat.

-Eat exotic sounding foods like quinoa, Sriracha, kale and broccoli. They're wonder foods.

-Fasting in the morning can help you lose weight.

Whew! These are only some of the myths that keep doing the rounds of the Internet and papers. People fall headlong for such untested and unscientific statements made by people who haven't the faintest clue what they're harking on about.

Agreed, a proper diet goes a long way in determining your health. In fact, six packs are not made at the gym; they are made in the kitchen. What you put into your mouth is equally important as what you lift at the gym. If your diet consists of junk food, fried food, foods with empty calories, and apart from the gym or the one hour exercise session at home, you lead a largely sedentary lifestyle, no matter how much you lift or how much time you spend exercising, the results will be disappointing. Studies have shown that people who were active throughout the day, walking here and there, carrying things, climbing stairs, cooking in the kitchen, playing with their children were much healthier on an average than someone who just went to the gym for a couple of hours and sat the whole day. The whole point of exercise and nutrition is to keep your body fit and functioning for a long span of time. Bad eating habits will soon nullify any good that you did at the gym.

Staying Healthy

Almost all nutritionists agree on certain principles for keeping the body healthy and sound.

1. Never Skip Breakfast-

Even if you're hard pressed for time, have a bowl of fruit and milk. Or brown bread with peanut butter. Skipping breakfast will cause hunger pangs later in the day, and you are more likely to munch unhealthy stuff like chips or wafers to combat the hunger. Have a hearty breakfast and watch your energy levels stay up all through the morning.

2. Go Easy on Fast Food-

There's no reason to give up on your favorite pizzas, burgers, fries and tacos. Just make sure you have them in a limited quantity at fixed time intervals. Say, once a month. Even better, make these at home. Then you'll have total control over the ingredients and can make healthier versions of pizzas and burgers right at home.

3. Eat Real Food-

This means food grown in a farm. Whole grains, rice, wheat, maize, corns, millets, beans, pulses, fruits, vegetables, nuts all constitute healthy and whole food. Eating homemade meals made of these will satiate your hunger, fill you with good calories and keep your metabolism active. Anything out of a box is a no-no. Focus on raw ingredients.

4. Drink, drink, drink-

By that, I mean water. Drink as much as you think you need. Forget about the 8-glasses rule or the 5-liter rule. Your body will tell you when it wants food and water. Drink and eat accordingly.

5. Eat Good Fats-

Eating fat won't make you fat. Nuts, butter, avocados all contain good fats that help your joints and muscles function smoothly and not clog your arteries. Eat them in a moderate amount, along with your stir-fries or cereal or just roasted.

6.Indulge occasionally-

There's absolutely no harm in eating a pastry or a rich caramel fudge or a wholesome homemade sweet made with butter or a tantalizing cheesy pizza or a heavenly tiramisu. But don't go overboard and ruin the hard work you put in all these months. Have these indulgences once in a while, say, once a month, and eat them in smaller portions. Savor each bite to get maximum satisfaction.

Conclusion

And finally here we are! By now you must have formed a pretty clear picture in your mind as to how you can control the weight gaining tendencies of your body the smart and regular practice of aerobics and by incorporating certain key components in your diet.

You would also be having a good idea as to how you can train with weights in the most efficacious manner by adopting certain key techniques that I have listed herein and by also performing the various exercises that I have mentioned. As a conclusion all I can tell you that gaining strength or endurance or size is not an overnight phenomenon. Hence make sure that your level perseverance and committed resilience never goes down.

Do not fall prey to the diet fads cropping up every day. Listen to your body; it is smarter than you think it is. Feed it good, wholesome food and exercise daily. You will remain healthy for a long time.

Your body is the only place you have to live in. Make it beautiful. Make it healthy. Start now.

Bonus

As my passion is sharing valuable information that tangibly impacts your life, I'd like to invite you to the free bonus below to positively affect your life in other dimensions, along with other tried and true methods I will send you.

If you want to take your health to the next level, I recommend the free resource below for some easy-to-follow quick tips that make a huge impact. *If you sign up, you will get the bonus immediately sent to your <u>valid</u> email address.*

Check the link below:

https://publishfs.leadpages.co/getultrahealth/

23 Health Tips & Hacks You Probably Aren't Doing But Should Be to Reduce Fatigue, Improve Sleep and Recovery, Boost Sex Drive, and Heal Your Gut

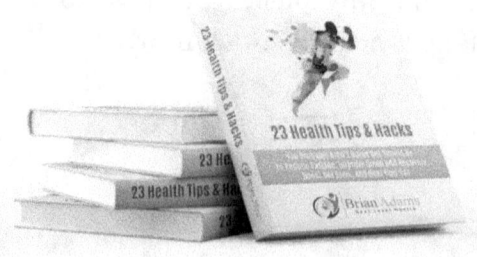